C0-AON-952

Dedication

Patricia Prince's

Cookbook
for
Optimum
Health

Compiled by
Patricia Prince
Sandra Prince Gwyn
Ellen Beck Prince

PERMISSION TO REPRINT MATERIAL FROM THIS BOOK MUST BE OBTAINED IN WRITING FROM THE AUTHOR.

FOR INFORMATION, WRITE:

Patricia Prince
Rt.3, Box 297
Mexia, TX 76667

FOURTH EDITION

©Copyright 1995, 1989, 1984, 1979 by E.S.P., Inc.

Lc. C.C. No. 79-89609
ISBN 0-8159-5221X

i

This book is dedicated to my two brothers
Joe and Benny Lucas
for their love and dedication; for their emotional and spiritual support, and for loving me as I am.

Thank you both for making it possible for me to enjoy the "Good Life."

About
The Author

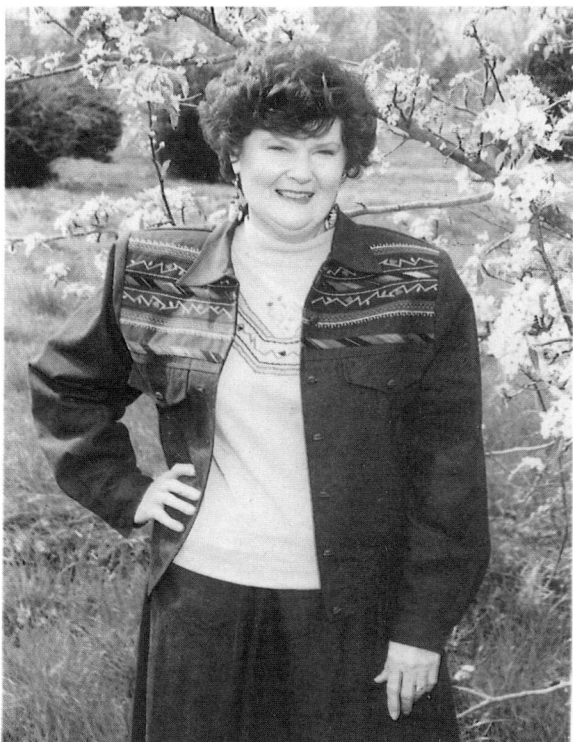

PHOTO BY: LILES, MEXIA, TEXAS

Patricia Prince

This book is composed of the philosophy of a better you. The author has devoted two and one-half hears of learning and diligent study of the aspects of Laetrile and the natural food diet. Through this book she has found a way to express herself in love and in the manner of well-being for her friends. This book is specially designed for you, and me; people searching for a plateau high above this present world, a plateau filled with inner peace and a special respect for yourself. In order for her to survive she must live with Laetrile as her closest companion and keep God in unity with herself and others. You see, I know this special lady, and through this book I hope you can gain what she has ...for this woman is Patricia Prince, my mother.

by Lee Wayne Prince
1979

Acknowledgements

ACKNOWLEDGEMENTS

There are so many people who influenced me in the writing of this book I could not possibly mention them all, but I feel I must introduce you to the ones without whom it would have been impossible.

My daughter, Sandra Prince Gwyn and my daughter-in-law, Ellen Beck Prince have worked untiringly research-ing, trying out recipes, mailing, writing letters and generally doing all the physical work involved in printing a book. My son, Lee Wayne Prince, did all the art work on the title pages. Also, my husband Calvin Prince, who stood beside me in the dark hours.

An
Approach
To
Cancer

Since I was first placed on the laetrile diet in April, 1977, it has been a constant problem to prepare meals. Every recipe would have to be changed to adhere to the diet. Oh, I could buy a book about some aspect of the Laetrile therapy with a few recipes thrown in the back, but who wants to cook from the back of some book?

I finally decided to compile a book of recipes that would be healthful and appetizing at the same time.

We all realize that the diet plays a very important role in correcting not only the underlying cause of cancer, but all degenerative diseases. Most of our lives we have lived to eat--now we must begin to eat to live. It is not easy to change your eating habits over night.

At first there will be withdrawal symptoms from all the additives, preservatives, caffeine, sugar, etc. that your body has been accustomed to receiving every day. But gradually you will notice that you are tasting food for the natural flavor and not for the seasoning added to it.

It is my desire that in some way this cookbook will assist you in following the laetrile diet and improve the "body" part of the holistic approach to your cancer.

Even though, as a cancer patient, my reasons for writing this book are to give other cancer patients a means to approach health, these recipes do fall within the confines of nutritional health for everyone.

As this book states over and over, it is very necessary that we eat as many raw foods as possible; fruits, vegetables, nuts, seeds and raw juices.

Since this is a "cook" book, naturally most of the recipes are for cooked foods. Raw food is best, steamed food is good, and cooked food or boiled food should be the third choice.

Just because it is for the Laetrile diet does not mean that all recipes may be used indiscriminately. For instance, if you have one of the health drinks with raw egg for breakfast, avoid all recipes containing egg for the rest of the day.

Also, be careful not to exceed the limits on such items as milk, cottage cheese and animal protein. If you use sea salt in one recipe, use sea salt the rest of the day.

Let the Modified Diet be your constant guide to eating.

Strict
Laetrile Diet

STRICT LAETRILE DIET

*(to be adhered to during the
first three weeks of detoxification
and intense Laetrile therapy)*

BEVERAGES
Herbal teas including chamomile, mint, papaya, comfrey.

FORBIDDEN
Alcohol, cocoa, coffee, soft drinks, pekoe and orange pekoe tea.

BREAD
Whole grain breads such as whole wheat, rye, bran muffins.

FORBIDDEN
White bread and products containing preservatives and refined flour.

CEREALS
Buckwheat, cornmeal, cracked wheat, millet, oats (oatmeal), fine ground grits.

FORBIDDEN
Processed cereals and any containing preservatives.

DAIRY PRODUCTS
None

FORBIDDEN
Includes cheese, eggs, and milk.

DESSERT

Home-made items from list of permitted foods; fresh fruits, unflavored gelatin.

FORBIDDEN

Others

FATS

Cold-pressed vegetable oils; <u>unsalted</u> butter in <u>limited</u> amounts.

FORBIDDEN

Animal fats and <u>hydrogenated</u> oils and margarine.

FISH

Very fresh only; preferably white fish.

FORBIDDEN

Other fish and sea foods.

FRUITS

Fresh fruits and unsulphured dried fruits.

FORBIDDEN

Canned, sweetened, or artificially preserved.

GRAINS

Fresh whole grains, such as millet, wheat, brown rice, flax seed.

FORBIDDEN

Not fresh, processed, etc.

JUICES
Only fresh fruit and vegetable juices.

FORBIDDEN
Canned, etc.

MEAT
Lean, grilled, broiled, roasted, or baked beef, chicken (without skin), lamb, turkey, and veal. Internal organs: heart and extra fresh calf liver.

FORBIDDEN
Pork and smoked or fat fried meats.

NUTS
Fresh, raw, untreated nuts.

FORBIDDEN
Roasted, salted, smoked, or flavored nuts.

POTATOES
Baked or boiled.

FORBIDDEN
Other forms (including potato chips).

SALADS
From fresh, raw vegetables, especially carrots, cauliflower, celery, chicory, green pepper, lettuce, radishes, swiss chard, watercress, onions, ripe tomatoes, turnips, brussels sprouts, broccoli.

FORBIDDEN
Vegetables which are not fresh.

SEASONINGS
Chives, garlic, onion, parsley, marjoram, sage, thyme, savory, cumin, oregano, laurel, herbs, capsicum (cayenne).

FORBIDDEN
Black pepper, paprika, sodium salt, and irritating spices.

SOUP
From fresh vegetables only.

FORBIDDEN
Canned, creamed, and from fat stock; consomme.

SWEETS
Unpasteurized honey, unsulphured molasses, raw sugar (yellow D) carob.

FORBIDDEN
Candy, chocolate, white sugar and refined sugar products.

VEGETABLES
Fresh, raw or fresh frozen, slightly cooked.

FORBIDDEN
Canned.

Modified
Laetrile Diet

MODIFIED LAETRILE DIET

BEVERAGES
Herbal teas including chamomile, mint, papaya, comfrey.

FORBIDDEN
Alcohol, cocoa, coffee, soft drinks, pekoe and orange pekoe tea.

BREAD
Whole grain breads such as whole wheat, rye, bran muffins.

FORBIDDEN
White bread and products containing preservatives and refined flour.

CEREALS
Buckwheat, cornmeal, cracked wheat, millet, oats (oatmeal_ fine ground grits.

FORBIDDEN
Processed cereals and any containing preservatives.

DAIRY PRODUCTS
In limited quantities, buttermilk, non-fat milk, non-fat cottage cheese, yogurt (preferably from a "Certified Raw Milk" dairy); poached or boiled egg, one per day.

FORBIDDEN
All others.

DESSERT

Home-made items from list of permitted foods; fresh fruits, unflavored gelatin and home-made sherbet from fresh ingredients.

FORBIDDEN
Others

FATS

Cold-pressed vegetable oils and unsalted raw butter.

FORBIDDEN
Animal fats and hydrogenated oils and margarine.

FISH

Very fresh only; preferably white fish.

FORBIDDEN
Other fish and sea foods.

FRUITS

Fresh fruits and unsulphured dried fruits.

FORBIDDEN
Canned, sweetened or artificially preserved.

GRAINS

Fresh whole grains, such as millet, wheat, brown rice, flax seed.

FORBIDDEN
Not fresh, processed, etc.

JUICES
Only fresh fruit and vegetable juices.

FORBIDDEN
Canned, etc.

MEAT
Lean, grilled, broiled, roasted or baked beef, chicken (without skin), lamb, turkey, and veal. Internal organs; heart and extra fresh calf liver.

FORBIDDEN
Pork and smoked or fat fried meats.

NUTS
Fresh, raw, untreated nuts.

FORBIDDEN
Roasted, salted, smoked or flavored nuts.

POTATOES
Baked or boiled.

FORBIDDEN
Other forms (including potato chips)

SALADS
From fresh, raw vegetables, especially carrots, cauliflower, celery, chicory, green pepper, lettuce, radishes, swiss chard, watercress, onions, ripe tomatoes, turnips, brussels sprouts, broccoli.

FORBIDDEN
Vegetables which are not fresh.

SOUP
From fresh vegetables only.

FORBIDDEN
Canned, creamed, and from fat stock; consomme.

SWEETS
Unpasteurized honey, unsulphured molasses, raw sugar (yellow D), carob.

FORBIDDEN
Candy, chocolate, white sugar and refined sugar products.

VEGETABLES
Fresh, raw or fresh frozen, slightly cooked.

FORBIDDEN
Canned.

Protein

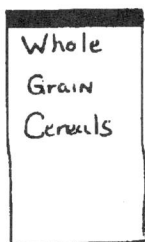

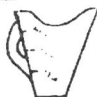

Whole Grain Cereals

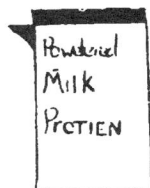

Powdered Milk Protien

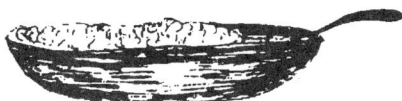

There is quite a controversy among Laetrile supporters concerning animal protein. Some doctors allow none whatsoever while some have no restrictions. Alternative doctors allow 3 1/2 ounces of animal protein a day from fish, chicken (without skin), beef or lamb, and one teaspoon of raw butter a day for seasoning. However, the animal proteins should be rotated day by day. Never eat the same animal protein two days in a row.

The following information is for those of you who are strict vegetarians and also for the meat eaters on the days you do not have meat. No vegetable by itself contains all the amino acids necessary to constitute a complete protein. Vegetables, grains and seeds must be combined properly in order to get the proper combinations. The following is a chart of the different foods that can be combined so that all the amino acids are present.

You will notice Soy Beans are missing from the list. Soy Beans are forbidden because they are an inferior protein and very had on the digestive system.

21

Grams Complete
Protein

Sesame

1/2 cup seeds +
   1/3 cup beans   =   19
1/4 cup seeds +
   1 cup milk   =   31
1/3 cup seeds +
   1 cup brown rice   =   16

Beans

1/4 cup +
   1 cup corn   =   14
1/2 cup +
   1 cup milk   =   22
1/4 cup +
   3/4 cup brown rice   =   15

Wheat

1 1/2 cup berries +
   1/2 cup beans   =   46
1 cup macaroni +
   1/4 cup cottage cheese   =   28

Milk

1 cup +
   1 medium potato   =   9

Rice

1 cup +
   1/4 cup Brewer's yeast   =   24
3/4 cup +
   1/4 cup cottage cheese   =   17
3/4 cup +
   1/3 cup instant milk   =   17

Try these combinations also:

Beans and seeds; mashed garbanzo and sesame seeds spread on whole wheat bread is very good. Also, split pea soup with sesame crackers. Black beans and brown rice or bean tostados or bean tacos are very tasty.

Try garbanzo sprouts, mixed nuts and beans as a salad.

Any grain with milk gives a complete protein. Also, mix beans plus nuts, plus milk at any meal.

Enjoy lentil soup made with milk. Also, sesame seeds or walnuts mixed in cottage cheese. Add sprouts to any meal to increase the protein.

Alternative doctors recommend powdered milk protein over the powdered vegetable protein because even though the protein from milk is from an animal source it is easier on the digestive system and uses less vital enzymes than the soy protein present in most powdered vegetable protein. If you can find a powdered or liquid protein without soy, that would be your best buy.

A
Few
Hints

HINTS

- All enzymes are destroyed at 130 degrees. Never heat oil over 240 degrees as it becomes toxic to the body.

- Anytime non-fat powdered milk is mentioned in this book, it is intended to be measured after it is mixed with water.

- Zucchini milk may be substituted for milk in any recipe. Just pare the zucchini, then run it through the blender (seeds and all). It can also be frozen for later use.

- Use yeast from health food stores which has no preservatives.

- One egg a day is allowed on the modified diet, so keep this in mind when using recipes containing eggs in any form.

- Salt – Sea salt is allowed in moderation. Try to gradually eliminate salt from your diet altogether. If you eat enough raw foods and juices, you will naturally get all the sodium your body needs.

- Steam vegetables over chicken broth to enhance their flavor.

- Add 1/2 teaspoon granulated or 500 ml. crushed Vitamin C to whole wheat bread recipes and they will be lighter and fluffier.

- Sliced fresh radishes may be substituted for canned water chestnuts in any recipe. They are also very tasty in soups or stews. Try them!

- Sprouted beans don't cause intestinal gas.

- Do not save oil and reheat it as it can develop carcinogenic properties in the process.

- Carob may be substituted for an equal amount of cocoa; or 3 tablespoons of carob powder is the same as 1 square of chocolate.

- When cooking beans, always add an acid-containing ingredient such as orange juice or tomatoes after simmering. Otherwise, the beans will be tough since acid slows down the softening process.

- As sprouts develop, nutritional content skyrockets. Vitamin C develops, Vitamin B multiplies, fat-soluble Vitamins A, D, E, and K increase. Many sprouts become complete proteins able to sustain life. Sprouts have all the minerals, enzymes, and still unknown factors necessary to the utilization of our food.

- Alcohol is not the only thing that destroys the liver and kidneys. Just as harmful are starches such as white bread, pastries, and candy; coffee and teas other than herbal teas also destroy the kidneys and liver.

- Cakes made with honey retain their moisture longer than cakes made with sugar.

- Just sprinkling a little dressing or lemon juice over raw vegetables on a bed of sprouts makes an excellent easy salad.

HINTS FOR COTTAGE CHEESE

- Sprinkle granola on cottage cheese for a delicious dessert.

- Mix cottage cheese with mashed avocado and a dash of lime or lemon juice. Serve with slices of melon.

- Garnish cottage cheese with chopped green onions, chives, fresh dill, parsley, pimento, green or black olives. Serve as a dip with crisp raw vegetables.

- Cottage cheese makes deviled egg filling much lighter and creamier.

- Try cottage cheese instead of whipped cream on gelatin desserts.

- Serve tea breads with a cottage cheese spread flavored with chopped dates or raisins and a dash of cinnamon or nutmeg.

NOTES ON DISTILLED WATER

Distilled water should not be used for all purposes. It is allowable to use any bottled water. This bottled water usually contains minerals which your body needs. You may also drink fresh well water or spring water as long as it has not been contaminated.

SOME NOTES ABOUT FATS

Just about every magazine and newspaper we pick up these days has an article about the dangers of saturated fats in our diets. As a result of these articles many people have tried to improve their health by cutting fats completely from their diets. As usually happens when we cut a nutrient completely we soon develop problems in that area. When any essential nutrient is totally cut out the body goes on red alert and starts to hoard that substance in various tissues and other areas of the body in order to have it for future use. An example of this is water retention; many times water retention is caused from the person not drinking enough water so the body starts to store it in the feet and legs and then around the heart. There are many instances where water retention is alleviated simply by having the person drink plenty of water. As soon as the body discovers that the water will be in continual supply it will begin to throw off the excess and the problem is solved.

So it is with fats. There are Essential Fatty Acids that the body needs to survive. Various research has shown that the Essential Fatty Acids may be acquired by having proper amounts of Extra Virgin Olive Oil and Flax Seed Oil in our diets. Dr. Budwig in Germany was nominated seven times for the Nobel Prize in Medicine for her research on Flax Seed Oil. Her research showed that laboratory animals that had all of the fats removed from their diets for a certain period of time showed an accumulation of fat around their hearts and cholesterol in the blood vessels. The control animals on the same diet only with the addition of flax seed oil showed a complete absence of fat buildup around the heart and no more than normal amounts of cholesterol in the blood.

The secret is to cut out completely the bad fats and oils and include Extra Virgin Olive Oil and Flax Seed Oil in your diet. Also, if other oils are used BE SURE THAT THEY ARE COLD PRESSED. This means that the oil was pressed out of the grains at a temperature below 110 degrees. And remember that to help maximize proper absorption and utilization of the Essential Fatty Acids and these good oils you MUST AVOID using hydrogenated and refined oils, margarine, and shortening, which contain Trans Fatty Acids. Moderate amounts of raw butter are allowed because it is a natural oil and in recent research has proved to be much better than margarine, which is one step removed from plastic in its manufacturing process.

Herbs

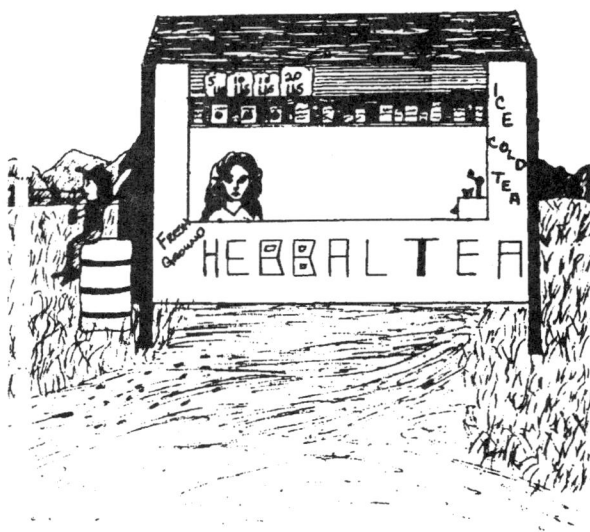

HERB TEAS

Are you "hung up" on coffee, teas, carbonated drinks, an occasional alcoholic drink, etc.? FORGET IT!! Try the herb teas instead. Just as you had to develop a taste for all those other beverages you will also have to develop a taste for herb teas. The first time I tasted an herb tea I almost gagged! But, I had decided to go all the way with this therapy so I tried again. The second cup wasn't so bad. Then the herb teas began tasting better. As I began to study herbs and their functions in the body, I began to realize that while I was having my tea in the place of other things, I was also healing my body. That encouraged me to try more of these wonderful herbs. For so long a time we have had the habit of reaching for a pill at the first symptom of discomfort; aspirin for headache, tranquilizers for nerves, Pepto Bismo for upset stomach, etc., and on and on. Now, when I feel a headache coming on I brew a cup of mint tea, valerian or comfrey for nervousness, spearmint for upset stomach.

This chapter is not intended to be a medical guide for ailments. The suggestions listed are those recommended by doctors who treat with herbs. As always, you should consult your doctor for any persistent symptom. Just enjoy the new taste of herbs and in doing so, you will naturally feel better. I just drink several cups of comfrey or chamomile tea a day for fun. Guests love lemon or mint teas. Try them!! You can buy all of these teas in your health food store.

Alfalfa Leaf - Stimulates kidneys, bowels, appetite, and aids digestion. Contains all the known vitamins and such minerals as Calcium, Magnesium, Phosphorous, and Potassium.

Alfalfamint - Vitamins and minerals. Arthritic conditions. Digestion. Alkalinizing.

Blue Violet - Lymph gland drainage. Healing sores. Severe coughs. Nasal drainage.

Catnip - Diaphoretic and tonic. Relaxes nerves. Good for colds.

Chamomile - Aids digestion. Clears complexion. Calms nerves and tensions. Constipation.

Comfrey (leaves and roots) - Heals tissues and eases pain. Removes toxic materials from the body. Loosens colds.

Cornsilk - Bladder and kidney. Genito-urinary tract. Mucous linings. Contains magnesium.

Dandelion - Contains iron to purify blood. Good for colds, dyspepsia, diabetes, rheumatism, arthritis, kidneys, gall bladder, liver. Contains calcium.

Elderberry - Colic, diarrhea, ovarian disturbances, builds blood.

Flaxseed - Constipation. Contains vitamin "F".

Golden Seal - Speeds up gastric juices by aiding digestion. Helps all mucous membrane problems. Colitis. Increases potency of other herbs.

Huckleberry - Good for high blood pressure, diarrhea, diabetes. Aids in digestion of starches.

Juniper - Bad breath, weak stomach, kidney, blood cleansing, and liver.

Papaya - Digestion of protein; aids dyspepsia, stomach weakness, pyorrhea.

Parsley - Excellent diuretic, good for gallstones, diabetes, jaundice. Contains iron and magnesium.

Peppermint - Aids digestion, circulation of blood, eliminates toxins. Contains manganese.

Raspberry - Tones female organs, good for circulation.

Rose Hips - High in vitamin C. Helps kidney functions.

Sage - Clears complexion, cleanses system. Sedative. Good for heart, liver, and kidneys.

Sassafras - Purifies blood, spleen, liver.

Sasparilla - Blood purifier. Good for rheumatism. Contains iodine.

Senna - Purgative, cleanses digestive tract, relieves constipation.

Spearmint - Diuretic. Nausea, vomiting. Contains iron.

Strawberry - Blood purifying. Diuretic. Heals mucus membranes. Contains sodium and iron.

White Oak - Diarrhea, dysentery, bowel problems. Contains iodine and potassium.

Lemon Grass - Cleanses tissues. Just a delicious tea to serve guests.

HERBS AS SEASONINGS

You can use herbs for seasoning and thereby cut down or eliminate the need for salt and pepper altogether. Black pepper is definitely a no-no on the diet, also paprika and irritating spices. Alternative doctors allow some of the aromatic spices, such as cinnamon, allspice, and nutmeg occasionally. But, they should be used with much discretion. You can buy Spike and Vegit in any health food store. Spike is a combination of herbs with a little sea salt added. Vegit is a combination of powdered vegetables with no salt whatsoever. They are both very delicious. When I first started using herbs, I had no idea which herbs to use with which vegetable or meat and as a result concocted a lot of inedible combinations. I found a list one day of different foods and the herbs best suited to them. I am including it in the book after eliminating the herbs not allowed on the diet.

Tomato or Vegetable Soup - Marjoram, Savory, Mixed herbs, Bay leaves.

Onion Soup - Thyme, Bay leaves, Parsley.

Chicken Soup - Parsley, Bay Leaves.

Broiled or Baked Fish - Basil, Marjoram.

Chopped Beef - Basil, Thyme, Allspice, Spike.

Stews - Thyme, Spike, Allspice, Bay Leaves, Oregano.

Filet Mignon - Spike.

Roast Beef - Thyme, Savory, Spike.

Stuffing for Chicken or Fowl - Marjoram, Thyme, Sage.

Eggplant - Oregano, Spike, Garlic.

Peas - Basil, Thyme.

Beans - Basil, Oregano, Garlic, Thyme.

Tomato - Basil, Marjoram, Sage, Spike.

Spinach - Marjoram.

Onions - Thyme, Spike.

Lima Beans - Savory.

Mushrooms - Marjoram.

Squash - Marjoram, Mint.

Carrots - Thyme, Mint.

Vegetable Salad - Spike, Garlic, Oregano, Basil.

Green Salad - Basil, Marjoram, Spike.

Salad Dressing - Basil.

Chicken Salad - Parsley, Marjoram.

Cottage Cheese - Sage, Spike, Marjoram.

Tomato Sauce - Basil, Oregano, Spike, Garlic.

Sprouts

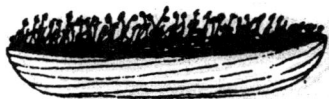

SPROUTS

Now don't turn up your nose at the sound of sprouts! They will open up a whole new world of flavor to you. They are very convenient to grow, and as the seed sprouts, vitamins C, B, A, D,E, and K are increased and many become complete proteins. Sprouts contain all the minerals and enzymes needed to sustain life. We need all the enzymes we can get and sprouts are one of our best sources.

Sprouts can be used in fresh salad, on breakfast cereal, in scrambled eggs, sprinkled on soups, in meat loaves, in breads, cupcakes, in health drinks, in sandwiches, fruit salads, or as a snack and in place of lettuce in winter.

Chop wheat, rye, alfalfa, or sunflower seed sprouts and add to any bread dough. Work into dough during last kneading. Use one cup of sprouts to every two cups liquid in the recipe. You can buy a sprouter in any health food store and go by the directions included, or if you prefer, grow sprouts as follows: Place 1 to 3 tablespoons of seeds in a quart jar and cover with water. One tablespoon of the small seeds and 3 tablespoons of large seeds. The next morning, drain the water off. Save this water to cook vegetables or rice as it contains some nutrients. Cover the jar with 2 layers of cheesecloth and lean bottom side up to let all the water drain off. Cover with a towel to keep seeds dark. Rinse seeds two or three times a day.

Wheat and lentils should not be sprouted longer than the

bean itself. Store in refrigerator and use in salads. Alfalfa and small seed sprouts will take about 5 days to get around 3 inches high. When 2 tiny leaves appear on alfalfa, uncover and place in the sun till they turn green. Then they are full of chlorophyll. Harvest and store tightly covered in refrigerator. Use these sprouts in <u>everything</u>.

SEED SPROUTING GUIDE
(Adapted from the Kitchen Garden People)

Variety of Seed	Hours Soaking Time	Times Daily Rinse	Days to Harvest	Suggested Uses
Alfalfa	8		3	3-4	Salads, Sandwiches, Juices
Beets	8		3	3-5	Salads, Juices
Chinese Cabbage	8		3	3-4	Salads, Juices
Corn	8		3	2-4	Tortillas, Vegetable Casseroles, Soups, Etc.
Dill	8		3	3-5	Salads, Sandwiches, Juices
Garbanzo	8		3	3-4	Vegetable Casseroles and Soups
Lentil	8		3	2-4	Salads, Juices, Vegetable Casserole, Soups, etc.

Variety of Seed	Hours Soaking Time	Times Daily Rinse	Days to Harvest	Suggested Use
Millet	8	3	3-5	Salads, Juices, Vegetable Casseroles, Soups, etc.
Peas, Alaskan	8	3	3-4	Salads, Soups, Omelets, Snacks
Peas, Special	8	3	3-4	Salads, Soups, Omelets, Snacks
Pichi Bean	8	3	3-5	Salads, Soups, Omelets, Oriental Dishes, Snacks
Porridge Pea	8	3	3-4	Salads, Soups, Oriental Dishes, Snacks

Variety of Seed	Hours Soaking Time	Times Daily Rinse	Days to Harvest	Suggested Uses
Radish	8	3	3-4	Sandwiches, Salads Juices
Red Clover	8	3	3-5	Sandwiches, Salads, Juices
Rye	8	3	2-3	Breads, Granola, Snacks
Sesame	8	3	2-3	Breads, Granola, Snacks
Triticale	8	3	1-2	Breads, Snacks, Granola, Pancakes
Wheat	8	3	2 days or wheat grass 5-7 days	Breads, Snacks, Granola, Pancakes

Raw Vegetable Juices

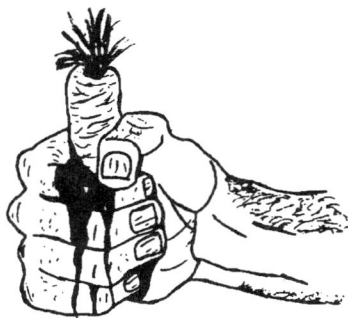

RAW VEGETABLE JUICES

As cancer patients, we have a battle on our hands to regain and to maintain the proper balance of our health. In order to do this, most of the food we eat must contain "life" or live, organic elements. These are found in fresh raw vegetables and fruits, seeds and nuts.

The quickest and easiest way to take advantage of these nutrients is to drink raw juices. Solid food takes hours to digest, but pure juices are very quickly digested, sometimes in a matter of minutes. This is done with very little exertion on the digestive system. Since many cancer patients either have very little appetite or have a hard time digesting raw food when they first begin metabolic therapy, raw juices are the best way we can furnish all the cells and tissues of the body with all the nutrients they need, and in a manner in which they can be quickly digested and absorbed. They build and regenerate the body because they contain all the amino acids, minerals, salts, vitamins, and enzymes needed by the body. That is, if they are fresh, raw, and no preservatives have been added. The toxic sprays used on vegetables are trapped in the fibers and are not present in the fresh juice.

It is well known, but not well publicized, that people who live entirely on fresh, raw foods, supplemented with lots of fresh vegetable and fruit juices, do not develop cancer.

I am not intimating that such a drastic change to raw foods

and juices does not require a certain amount of intestinal fortitude, especially for those of us accustomed to a diet of 90 or 95 percent cooked or processed foods. I am not suggesting that anyone go on a strict raw diet altogether. Alternative doctors advocate some cooked food - as it is their assumption that a certain amount of cooked food is beneficial to our well being. We should include as much raw food as we feel we can tolerate in our diet.

The very fact that you are reading this book tells me that you have an earnest desire to improve your lifestyle. Correcting bad eating habits is the best place to start, since eating a proper diet will furnish the body with all the live elements we so desperately need to control cancer.

There is quite a bit of controversy among those who are supposed to know about which kind of juicer is best to extract juices from fruits and vegetables. The hydraulic press seems to get the most votes. However, hydraulic presses are very expensive. Most experts seem to agree that the centrifugal type of juicer is suitable if it is not allowed to heat up. The heat will destroy the enzymes. All juices should be drunk immediately, to get the most benefit from the enzymes and other nutrients. Until your body becomes accustomed to the juices, it would be a good idea to dilute them up to 1/2 with distilled water. When different juices are combined, the proportion of elements in each juice is changed to correspond with similar elements in the other juices, giving a totally different formula. The effects of these combinations is of great importance to the healing of the body. The combinations of some of these juices are listed at the end of this chapter. I have listed some of the most popular juices along with some of their nutritional value. As with the chapter on herb teas, this chapter is not intended to be a prescription of treating certain ailments. The values of the juices for certain malfunctions in the body are suggestions I have come across in my research which included books and articles written by various authorities on the subject.

BEET JUICES
Helps to build up red corpuscles in the blood. Start out drinking beet juice by combining 3 ounces with 1 pint carrot juice. Gradually add more beet juice. If taken alone, when you are not used to it, the cleansing effects of beet juice on the liver may cause a slight nausea. Contains calcium, potassium, chlorine, and sodium.

When beet juice is combined with carrot juice, they give phosphorous, sulphur, and a very high content of Vitamin A.

CABBAGE JUICE
There have been numerous fantastic responses to cabbage juice in treating duodenal ulcers. It has wonderful cleansing and reducing properties. Sometimes causes intestinal gas formed when the cleansing elements of the juice begin to dissolve waste matter. Enemas help remove both the gas and waste and the result is a new feeling of health.

Cabbage juice is loaded with sulphur, chlorine, and iodine. When added to carrot juice, the result is an excellent form of Vitamin C. Cabbage juice is very effective in relieving constipation. Adding salt to cabbage or its juice destroys its value.

CARROT JUICE

One of the richest sources of carotene, which turns to Vitamin A in the body. It also contains Vitamins B, C, D, E, G, and K, and a good supply of calcium, magnesium, iron, phosphorous, sulphur, silicon, and chlorine.

It is especially helpful in normalizing the whole system, promotes appetite and aids digestion, and aids in dissolving ulcers and cancer. Always cut off tops of carrots 1/2 inch below the ring where the green stem starts. Add a little raw goat's milk for an exotic flavor.

CELERY JUICE

Contains "organic" sodium and calcium in the proper quantities to afford the proper utilization of calcium in the body. Especially helpful in repairing damage done by years of consumption of concentrated sugars and starches such as breads, biscuits, cakes, cereals, doughnuts, spaghetti, etc. It is a natural body "air conditioner". It is both soothing and comforting during extremely hot weather to have a glass of fresh raw celery juice mid-afternoon. It normalizes the body temperature to the extent that you will be perfectly comfortable while those around you are complaining of the heat. Also very high in magnesium and iron, hence it helps in feeding the blood cells.

CUCUMBER JUICE
Aids growth of nails and hair, helps regulate high and low blood pressure, and equally helpful in disturbances of teeth and gums. High in silicon and sulphur, also it is 40% potassium, 10% sodium, 7 1/2% calcium, 20% phosphorus, and 7% chlorine. Best when combined with other juices.

LETTUCE JUICE
Mixed with carrot and spinach juice, it furnishes food to the nerves and roots of the hair. When combined with carrot, green pepper, and alfalfa juice, it helps restore hair to its natural color. Contains more than 38% potassium, 15% calcium, more than 5% iron, and 6% magnesium. Lettuce also contains 9% phosphorus and an ample supply of sulphur and silicon.

Use the darker outside leaves and omit the lighter shade of leaves in the center, as the outer leaves contain more chlorophyll.

PAPAYA JUICE
I realize papaya is a fruit and not a vegetable, but I decided to include it as it is a very healthful food and the juice is such an aid to digestion. It contains papain, which has the same digestive effect as pepsin on the system. It is very helpful in the coagulation of clotting of blood. The green papaya has much more active enzymes than the ripe. In fact, it's healing process is so widely known, many people use it for the healing of most any digestive disorder.

PARSLEY JUICE

Parsley is not a vegetable. It is an herb and highly concentrated. Small amounts should always be mixed with either carrot or celery juice. Parsley juice has ingredients which are very helpful to oxygen metabolism. It also helps maintain the small blood vessels and the functioning of the kidneys and bladder. It is also helpful to the eyes and optic nervous system. Very high source of chlorophyll.

GREEN PEPPER JUICE

Contains an abundance of silicon. Helpful in clearing up skin blemishes when taken regularly with carrot juice. Also helps relieve gas in the alimentary canal.

TOMATO JUICE

Fresh, raw tomato juice is alkaline if drunk when no starches or sugars are eaten or drunk during the same meal. In combination with sugars or starches, the effect is definitely acid. Rich in sodium, calcium, potassium, and magnesium.

WATERCRESS JUICE

A very strong juice and should never be taken alone. When mixed with spinach juice and some lettuce and turnip leaf juice, the combination has the ability to assist in increasing oxygen transmission in the blood stream. Very high in sulphur, phosphorus, and chlorine. Contains 20% potassium, 18% calcium, 8% sodium, 5% magnesium, and 1/4 of 1% iron.

STRING BEAN JUICE
Furnishes a natural insulin which assists the pancreatic functions of the digestive system.

TUNRIP JUICE
Turnip leaves contain more calcium than any other vegetable. Also high in potassium, When combined with carrot and dandelion juice, the magnesium in the dandelion works with the calcium in the turnip leaves and the elements in carrots to give firmness and strength to the bone structure.

DANDELION JUICE
Obtain juice from leaves as well as the root. High in potassium, sodium, and calcium. Dandelion juice is our richest food in iron and magnesium content. Prevents softness of the bones and also gives strength and firmness to the teeth.

OXYGEN COCKTAIL
Handful watercress
1 cup spinach leaves
1 cup turnip leaves
1 cup lettuce leaves

These combinations of juices are very healthful in a variety of ways:

1. *Carrot, apple, beet
2. *Carrot, beet, celery
3. *Carrot, beet, cucumber

4. *Carrot, lettuce, beet
5. Celery, parsley, *carrot
6. Cucumber, *carrot
7. Green peppers, *carrot
8. *Carrot, orange
9. Spinach, parsley, cucumber, *celery
10. Brussels sprouts, string beans, *carrot
11. Cucumber, turnip, *celery
12. Watercress, parsnip, potato, *carrot

* Denotes larger portion of juice
NOTE: Use tops and roots of dandelion, turnips, radish, and beets.

Any vegetable or fruit juice combination which tastes good "to" you is also good "for" you. So use your imagination again for a whole new adventure in "drinking". Here are a few combinations to help you get started:

BLOOD STRENGTHENER
3 Carrots
2 Medium beets
2 Cups spinach

TO CLEAN THE BODY
3 Stalks celery
1 Cup cabbage
3 Medium carrots
1 Cup dandelion greens
1/2 Cup distilled water

RED DRINK

3 Stalks celery

2 Medium beets

3 Medium carrots

1 Cup parsley

CARROT - APPLE

1 Apple (seeds & peeling)

4 Medium carrots

GREEN DRINK

1 Cucumber

1 Green pepper

3 Stalks celery

2 Stalks broccoli

Handful parsley

Sounds terrible and looks terrible. Drink for several days in a row and you begin to like it!

DANDELION DELIGHT

1 Cup dandelion greens

1 Cup turnip leaves

3 Medium carrots

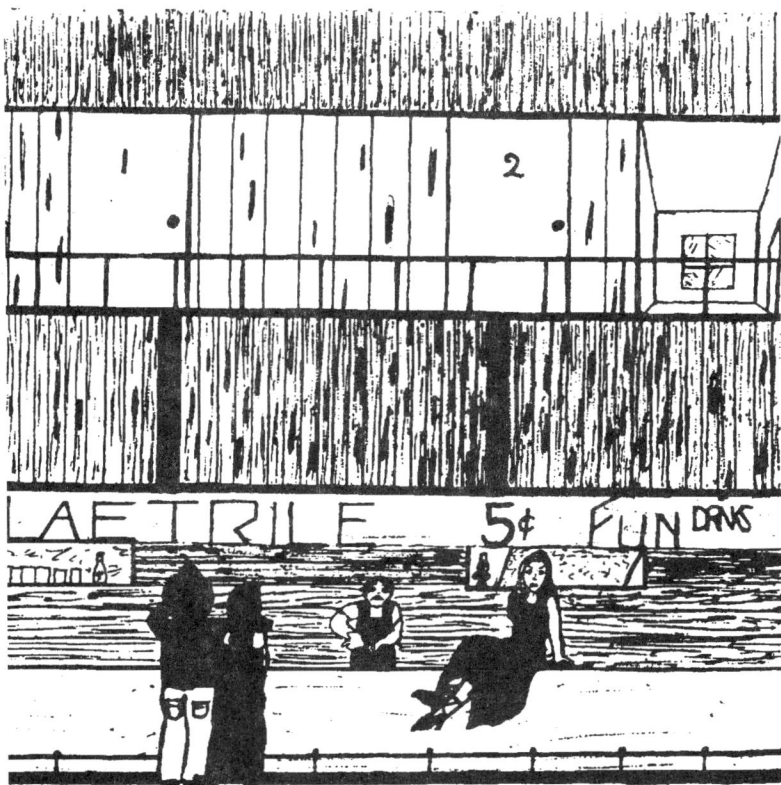

Fun Drinks

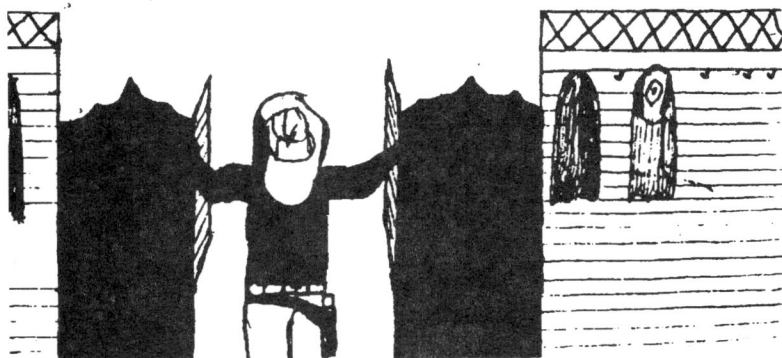

These drink recipes are what I call my fun drinks. They are so quick and easy to prepare. I usually drink any of the ones made with milk as my breakfast and find I have more energy.

Any of these drinks may be frozen - the milk ones are delicious to partially freeze and serve as a malt or freeze them and eat for ice cream. Freeze the others hard, then break into chunks, place back in the blender for half a minute and you have a delicious sherbet.

Experiment with different juices for a variety of drinks. Any fruit may be used in any of the recipes. With a little imagination, you can have a different drink every day of the year. Alternative doctors recommend the powdered milk protein above the powdered vegetable protein because most of the vegetable formulas contain soy protein which is not allowed on the diet. Soy protein is a very inferior protein and saps the body of enzymes that are vital to the cancer patient.

APPLE ENERGY

1 Cup fresh strawberries

1 Cup apple juice

1/2 Large banana

1 Tablespoon lecithin (granular)

1 Tablespoon powdered protein (milk)

1 Egg (optional)

1 Teaspoon honey (optional)

Blend 1 minute at high speed.

BANANA PICK-UP

1 Tablespoon lecithin (granular)

1 Tablespoon powdered protein (milk)

1 Cup non-fat milk

1 Large banana

1/4 Teaspoon pure vanilla

1 Teaspoon honey (optional)

Blend 1 minute at high speed.

APRICOT DELIGHT

Place in blender:

1 Cup diced fresh pineapple

1 Cup fresh raspberries (unsweetened)

1 Teaspoon unsulphured molasses

6 Pitted apricots

6 Apricot kernels

Blend till smooth and drink immediately.

LAETRILE COCKTAIL
1 Banana
1/2 Cup pure apple juice
1 Tablespoon brewer's yeast
1 Teaspoon apricot kernels
1/2 Teaspoon cinnamon
1 Tablespoon honey

Place all ingredients in blender and run at high speed for 1 minute. Drink at once.

VIM-N-VIGOR DRINK
1 Cup non-fat milk
1/2 Cup orange juice
1 Banana
2 Tablespoons wheat germ
1 Teaspoon honey

Blend well and serve.

APPLE JUICE PROTEIN DRINK
1 1/2 Cups apple juice
1 Tablespoon lecithin granules
1 Tablespoon powdered protein (milk)
1/2 Large banana
1 Raw egg

Blend in blender at high speed for 1 minute. Delicious energy drink for any time of day. Do not eat anything with egg in it on the day you drink a raw egg. This drink is also a good energy drink without the egg.

PROTEIN DRINK

1 Tablespoon powdered protein (milk)
1 1/2 Teaspoon granular lecithin
1 Cup fresh (or frozen unsweetened) strawberries
1 Raw egg
1 Cup non-fat milk

Blend. This drink can be made with any fruit for variations you like. Substitute yogurt for milk or leave out the egg and increase protein. Add honey, wheat germ or brewer's yeast for a different flavor. Add your Vitamin A to this drink, also.

VITAMIN C DRINK

Peel and section 1 orange, 1 lemon, 1 grapefruit and a small portion of each peel. Place in blender on liquify till you have a pale yellow puree. Sweeten with a little honey. Mix with equal parts distilled water. Serve hot or cold.

● ● ●

HOT CAROB

2 Tablespoons carob powder
1 Tablespoon honey
1/2 Teaspoon pure vanilla
1/8 Teaspoon sea salt
1/2 Cup water (distilled)
2 Cups non fat milk

Mix carob powder, honey, sea salt, and water in a small pan. Boil one minute stirring constantly. Lower heat and add milk. Heat well, but do not boil. Add vanilla. Serve hot.

CAROB SHAKE

Freeze above recipe and break into chunks in blender. Blend at high speed for 30 seconds. Just like a chocolate malt. Almost.

<u>QUICK ENERGY DRINK</u>
1/2 Cup alfalfa sprouts
1/2 Cup sunflower seeds
3 apples with skins and seeds, quartered
1 1/2 Tablespoons brewer's yeast
1 1/2 Tablespoons raw honey
1/2 cup non-fat milk
1/4 Cup wheat germ
Juice of 1 lemon
Liquify in blender.

Dressings, Sauces & Butters

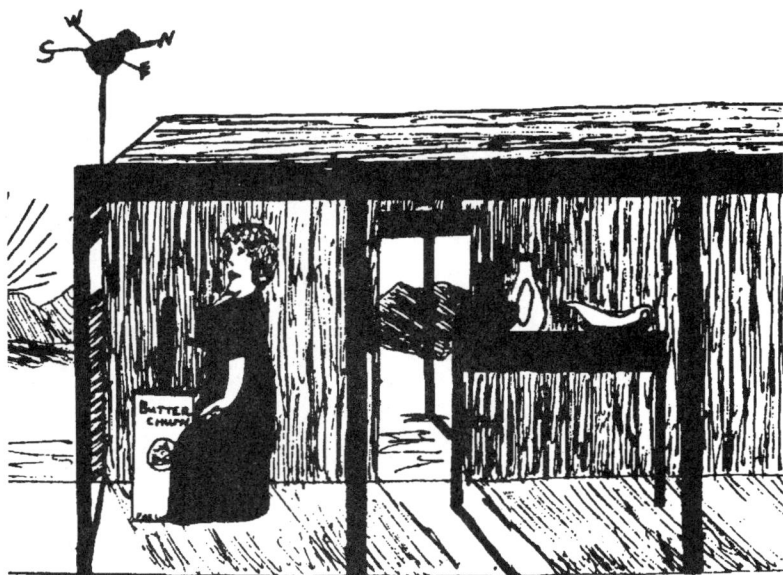

I was really surprised when I found out how many delicious dressings, sauces, and butters I could make in my blender. Dig around in the back of your cabinet and drag your blender out and put it to use. Also, use your imagination with these recipes to add herbs, chopped vegetables, onion, garlic, etc. Just as you can vary the juices and drinks with a "dab of this and a dash of that" you can create new flavors for almost all your foods. So "go creative" with this chapter!

MAYONNAISE

Place in blender:
1 Whole egg
2 Tablespoons lemon juice
1/2 Teaspoon sea salt

Start blender and add very slowly: 3/4 Cup cold pressed oil
Blend to desired consistency. For fruit salads add 2 Teaspoons honey to first three ingredients.

● ● ●

ONION DRESSING

Beat vigorously:
3/4 Cup cold pressed oil
1/2 Cup plus 1 tablespoon lemon juice
1 Teaspoon sea salt

Then add:
3 Tablespoons minced onion

● ● ●
Vegetable Salad Dressing

2 Tablespoons each: shredded carrot, celery, onion, and
  parsley
Garlic to taste
1 Teaspoon sea salt
1 3/4 Cup cold pressed oil
1/2 cup lemon juice

Place all ingredients in blender at high speed for 2 minutes.
Keep in covered jar in cool place. Gets better with age.
Use sparingly.

COTTAGE CHEESE DRESSING

8 Ounces non fat cottage cheese
3/4 Cup buttermilk
1/4 Cup apple cider vinegar
1 Teaspoon oregano
1/2 Teaspoon garlic powder
1 Teaspoon sea salt
1 Small onion, chopped finely

Blend cottage cheese till liquid. Pour into bowl and add rest of ingredients. Chill. Serve over fresh vegetables or fruit salads.

● ● ●

LEMON SALAD DRESSING

Beat:
1/2 Cup cold pressed oil
2 Tablespoons lemon juice
1/2 Teaspoon sea salt
1 Well beaten egg yolk

Make a smooth sauce in double boiler with:

1 Tablespoon cold pressed oil
2 Tablespoons whole wheat flour
1/2 Cup distilled water

Pour into first mixture and beat rapidly. Use sparingly.

FRUIT JUICE DRESSING

Blend:4 Tablespoons cold pressed oil
2 Tablespoons fresh lemon juice
6 Tablespoons fresh orange juice
2 Tablespoons fresh pineapple juice
2 Teaspoons warmed raw honey

Pour over fruit salad.

• • •

HONEY MINT SAUCE

1/2 Cup water (distilled)
1 Tablespoon lemon juice
1 Cup raw honey
1/4 Cup chopped mint

Heat water and lemon juice in top of double boiler. Stir in honey. Add mint and cook slowly for 5 minutes.

• • •

CRANBERRY RELISH

3 Ounces water (distilled)
2 Cups raw cranberries
1 Peeled and quartered orange
1 Small piece orange rind

Blend in blender until desired consistency. For a sweet relish add honey to taste.

HOMEMADE TOMATO SAUCE

2 Tablespoons oil
1 Chopped onion
5 Lbs. fresh tomatoes
1 Bay leaf
1/2 Teaspoon garlic powder
1/2 Teaspoon basil
1/2 Teaspoon marjoram
1/4 Teaspoon crushed fennel seed

Saute onion in oil (not over 240 degrees). Add chopped tomatoes and bay leaf. Simmer until thick. Add rest of ingredients and cook 10 more minutes. Store in refrigerator.

● ● ●

ITALIAN TOMATO SAUCE

4 Lbs. fresh tomatoes, quartered
2 Large diced carrots
4 Stalks diced celery
2 Diced onions
1 Small bunch chopped parsley

Cook slowly until thick (about 2 hours).
Blend until smooth and add:
3 Tablespoons olive oil

Return to pan and simmer another hour. Delicious served over whole wheat or zucchini spaghetti. This sauce may be stored by filling a jar pouring olive oil on top to keep air out. Keep in cool, dark place.

PARSLEY MAYONNAISE

1 Egg
2 Tablespoons lemon juice
1/2 Teaspoon dry mustard
1/2 Teaspoon sea salt
1/8 Teaspoon cayenne
1 Cup cold pressed oil
1/4 cup chopped parsley

Combine egg, lemon juice, salt substitute, cayenne, and 1/4 cup cold pressed oil in blender. Cover, turn to high speed, remove feeder cap and immediately begin pouring remaining oil into mixture in a slow stream. Process until thoroughly blended and smooth. Stir in parsley. Chill. Makes about 1 1/4 cups.

• • •

PARSLEY BUTTER

Cream 1/2 cup softened raw butter. Blend in 1 tablespoon snipped parsley, 1 teaspoon lemon juice, 1/2 teaspoon savory, and 1/4 teaspoon sea salt. Makes 1/2 cup. This is very good on potatoes.

ORANGE FRENCH DRESSING

3/4 Cup frozen concentrated, unsweetened orange juice, thawed and undiluted
1/2 Cup cold pressed oil
1/4 Cup apple cider vinegar
1/2 Teaspoon dry mustard
1/4 Teaspoon sea salt
1/8 Teaspoon tabasco sauce

ORANGE FRENCH DRESSING - Continued

Combine all ingredients and beat with electric mixer until blended. Cover and store in refrigerator. Shake well before serving. Makes 1 1/2 cups.

● ● ●

APPLE SYRUP

3 Cups unsweetened apple juice
2 Tablespoons raw butter
2 Tablespoons whole wheat flour

Boil juice down to 1 1/2 cup. Melt butter over low heat. Stir in flour. Gradually add juice, stirring constantly. Raise heat and simmer 5 minutes. Do not boil. Good for pancakes, biscuits, or spooned over plain cake.

HERB BUTTER

1/2 Cup raw butter softened
1 Tablespoon finely snipped fresh herb or 3/4 dried herb
1 Teaspoon lemon juice

Cream raw butter till fluffy. Crush dried herb with mortar and pestle. Combine herb and lemon juice with butter. Keep herb butter at room temperature for 1 hour to mellow. Store extra butter in refrigerator.

● ● ●

HERB BUTTER - FOR CORN

To 1/2 cup raw butter, add 1/2 teaspoon dried rosemary, crushed, and 1/2 teaspoon marjoram, crushed. Blend with a spoon till light and fluffy.

SESAME BUTTER

1 Cup sesame seeds
1 Tablespoon oil

Blend at high speed for 2 minutes.
Use as butter to season cooked vegetables.
Use as a spread for bread or crackers.

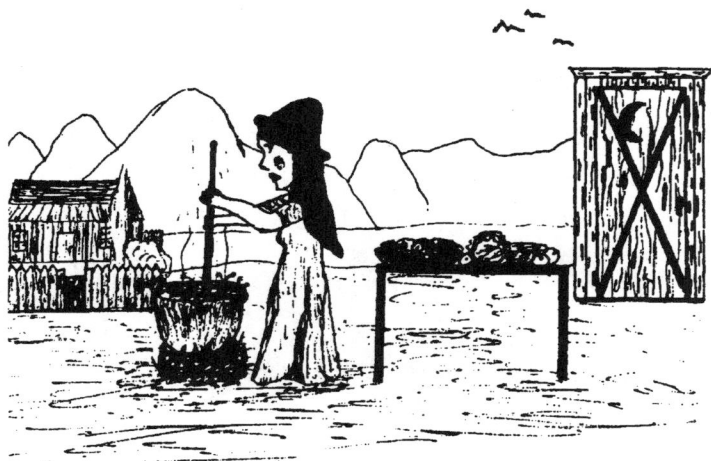

Soups & Salads

PLAIN CREAM OF CHICKEN SOUP

2 Cups chicken (without skin) broth
1 Cup water (distilled)
3 Tablespoons whole wheat flour
1/2 Cup non-fat milk powder

Use chicken (without skin) broth that has had all fat removed. Pour into saucepan. Stir powered milk and flour into water and simmer until creamy. Season with sea salt or Vegit or not at all.

● ● ●

CHICKEN CORN SOUP

3 to 3 1/2 lb. chicken (without skin)
6 Cups water (distilled)
1 Carrot, chopped
1 Onion, chopped
2 Tablespoons chopped parsley
1 1/4 Cups fresh or frozen corn
2 Cups whole wheat noodles
3 Hard boiled eggs (omit for strict diet)

Bring skinned chicken, water, carrot, onion, parsley, and celery to boil, then reduce heat and simmer about 1 hour and 15 minutes. Chicken should be tender. Remove chicken. Strain broth and put in refrigerator to congeal fat. Lift off fat. Cook whole wheat noodles according to directions on package. Remove chicken from bones and cut in large pieces. Return chicken to broth on medium heat, add corn, noodles, egg slices.

Bring soup to boil and serve hot. Serves 6 to 8.

LENTIL - MUSHROOM STEW

1 1/2 Quarts water
2 Cups lentils
1 Onion, sliced and chopped
1/2 Pound mushrooms, sliced
1 Teaspoon dried basil
1/2 Teaspoon sea salt
2 Stalks celery, chopped
2 Carrots, sliced
1/3 Cup cold pressed oil
2 Tablespoons cider vinegar

Slowly add the lentils to boiling water. Reduce heat to simmer and cook one hour. Saute onion, mushrooms, and basil in oil, being careful not to heat the oil over 240 degrees. Set aside. Combine all ingredients except vinegar and seasonings and cook 1 hour more or until lentils are tender. Add vinegar and seasonings before serving. Serves 5. Very good with grain dishes.

● ● ●

LENTIL SOUP

1 1/2 Cups lentils
1 1/2 Quarts water
1/2 Teaspoon sea salt
2 Stalks celery, chopped
1 Onion, chopped
1 Teaspoon tarragon
2 Carrots, diced
2 Tablespoons
 cold pressed oil
1 Tablespoon lemon
 juice

Place lentils in pot, add water and sea salt. Cover and simmer 1 hour. Add other ingredients. Cover and simmer 15 minutes. Serves 6.

POTATO SOUP

1/2 lbs. potatoes, diced (do not peel)
3 Leeks, white part only, diced
       (or 1/2 cup diced onion)
5 Cups distilled water
1 Clove garlic, minced
Juice of 1 lemon
Dash of cayenne
1 Tablespoon yeast extract
Sea salt to taste
1 Tablespoon minced leek tops
 (or 1 tablespoon dried parsley)
Plain yogurt (Natural, unsweetened)

Simmer first 6 ingredients 20 minutes or until potatoes are tender. Cool slightly and blend in blender. Stir in yeast. Add sea salt. Chill. Stir heaping tablespoon yogurt into each serving. May also be heated after chilled and served hot.

● ● ●

HINT: Use yogurt in baked potatoes to take the place of sour cream. Very good!!!!!

CHICKEN BROTH

3 1/2 lb. hen (without skin)
Celery, stalks and leaves
Whole onion
Carrot, washed and unpeeled
Bay leaf
Parsley

Place all ingredients in pot and cover with distilled water. Simmer on low heat for 2 hours. Remove vegetables and puree in blender; bone chicken (without skin) and cut in small pieces. Return everything to soup. Heat and serve.

COLD CUCUMBER SOUP

2 Medium cucumbers
1 Quart buttermilk
1 Tablespoon snipped green onion
1 Teaspoon sea salt
1/4 cup snipped parsley

Pare cucumbers, remove seeds, and grate to make 1 to 1 1/2 cups. Add the remaining ingredients; mix well. Cover and chill 1 hour. Be sure to mix again just before serving. Trim with parsley sprigs. Serves 8 to 10.

LENTIL BANANA SOUP

Cook lentils according to package directions seasoning with cold pressed oil and sea salt. Fifteen minutes before they finish cooking slice one or two bananas into the beans and allow to cook.

BEEF STOCK

6 Lbs. beef soup bones
        (have the butcher cut in pieces)
1 Cup chopped onion
1/2 Cup chopped celery
1 Large bay leaf
4 Sprigs parsley
2 Teaspoons sea salt

Place meat bones and 2 1/2 quarts distilled water in large sauce pan. Simmer uncovered (don't boil) 3 hours. Remove bones; cut off meat and chop. Return meat to stock; add remaining ingredients. Simmer uncovered 2 hours longer. Strain. Chill and lift off fat. Makes 6 cups. Use in all recipes calling for consomme or beef bouillon cubes.

CREAM OF MUSHROOM SOUP

1 Cup fresh mushrooms
2 Tablespoons chopped onion
2 Tablespoons whole wheat flour
2 Cups chicken (without skin) broth or beef stock
1/2 Cup non-fat milk
1/2 teaspoon sea salt
1/4 Teaspoon ground nutmeg

Slice mushrooms through cap and stem; cook with onion in 2 tablespoons raw butter five minutes. Blend in whole wheat flour; add chicken broth or beef stock. Cook and stir until slightly thickened. Cool slightly; add non-fat milk and seasonings. Heat through. Serve at once. Serves 4 to 6.

● ● ●

SPLIT PEA SOUP

1/2 Lb. green split peas
1 Cup chicken (without skin) stock
3/4 Cup sliced onion
1/8 Teaspoon dried marjoram, crushed
1 Cup diced celery
1 Cup diced carrots

Cover peas with 3 cups distilled water and the chicken stock. Simmer gently 2 minutes; remove from heat; cover and let stand one hour. Add onion, 1/2 teaspoon salt substitute and marjoram. Bring to a boil; cover, reduce heat, and simmer (don't boil) 1 1/2 hours. Stir occasionally. Add vegetables. Cook slowly, uncovered, 30 to 40 minutes. Serves 6 to 8.

CHICKEN NOODLE SOUP

3 to 3 1/2 lb. Chicken (without skin)
6 Cups cold water (distilled)
1 Small onion, chopped
1 Stalk celery, chopped
1 Carrot, chopped
1 Small parsnip, chopped
1 1/2 Cups whole wheat noodles

Bring water, skinned chicken, onion, celery, carrot, and parsnip to a boil. Then reduce to low heat and simmer 1 hour and 15 minutes. The chicken should not fall off the bones but should be tender. Remove chicken from the broth. Strain broth and put in refrigerator to congeal fat, lift off fat. Cook noodles according to package directions. Heat broth, add noodles and cook gently 1 minute. Then chop chicken and add to broth.

● ● ●

COLE SLAW

2 Cups shredded cabbage
1 Carrot, grated fine
1/3 Cup apple cider vinegar
2 Tablespoons honey
3 Teaspoons homemade mayonnaise

Mix vinegar, honey, and mayonnaise together; pour over cabbage and carrot; toss lightly. Serve at once.

COTTAGE CHEESE DELIGHT

Melt 2 tablespoons raw butter, add 3 tablespoons whole wheat flour, and gradually blend in 1 cup low-fat milk, mixing well. Cook over low heat until smooth and thick. Beat yolks of 2 eggs until light and lemon colored. Gradually beat in 1/3 cup honey, 1/2 teaspoon sea salt, and 2 teaspoons grated lemon or orange rind. Add 1/2 cup chopped raw almonds, 1/2 cup raisins, 1 cup cottage cheese and white sauce. Blend well. Beat egg whites until stiff but not dry and fold gently into cheese mixture. Butter generously a 1 1/2 quart casserole. Sprinkle thickly with fine dry whole wheat bread crumbs, reserving some for top. Pour in cheese mixture, sprinkling remainder of crumbs on top. Dust lightly with grated nutmeg. Place casserole in shallow pan of hot water. Bake in moderate oven at 350 degrees for 50 to 60 minutes until set, and top is brown. Serve warm with a fruit sauce.

Do not eat anything else with eggs on the day you eat this salad.

MACARONI SALAD

1 - 8 Ounce box elbow whole wheat
    or zucchini macaroni
1/2 Cup chopped fresh pimento
1 Chopped small onion
2 Stalks chopped celery
1/2 Chopped green pepper
1 Tablespoon sesame seeds
1/2 Teaspoon Vegit
1/2 cup homemade mayonnaise

Cook macaroni in distilled water according to directions on package. Drain. Mix in remaining ingredients. Serve on a bed of lettuce leaves and decorate with springs of parsley.

PRUNE SALAD

Cut up navel oranges, bananas, and pitted prunes that have been soaked to plump them. Top with cottage cheese or honey sweetened yogurt. Refrigerate leftovers.

TOSSED SALAD

Bibb lettuce
Boston lettuce
Iceberg lettuce
Romaine lettuce
Escarole
Chicory
Endive
Watercress
1 Clove garlic
3 Thin sliced radishes
1 Cucumber cut in chunks
1 Tomato, cut in cubes

Place radishes, cucumber, and tomato in bottom of large bowl. Chop greens and place on top. Peel garlic, put in garlic press and press over salad. Then add 1 tablespoon lemon juice. Toss greens lightly.

CUCUMBER SALAD

Combine:
1/2 Onion, peeled, ground, and drained
2 Cucumbers, peeled, ground, and drained
1 Tablespoon red wine vinegar
1 Teaspoon sea salt
1 Teaspoon honey
1 Clove garlic, crushed

Let ripen at least 6 hours before using. Serve on mixed greens or use mixture to stuff tomatoes.

CELERY SALAD

1 Celery stalk, diced
1 Unpeeled green apple, diced
1 Avocado, diced
1/4 Cup chopped cashews, almonds, walnuts

Toss all together, add your favorite dressing. Sprinkle with wheat germ. Remember to use raw nuts, always.

● ● ●

DELICIOUS RAW VEGETABLE SALAD

Combine 1/2 cup each of alfalfa sprouts, raw sliced mushrooms, raw cauliflower buds, green beans (steamed and chilled) with 1 head of Boston lettuce, torn in small pieces. Serve with lemon dressing.

● ● ●

HI-PROTEIN HEALTH SALAD

2 Cups wheat or alfalfa sprouts
1/3 Cup sunflower seeds
2 Apples, grated
2 Sliced bananas
1/3 Cup raisins
1/3 Cup plain natural yogurt

Mix and serve. Good for breakfast.

SALAD WITHOUT LETTUCE

1 Sliced cucumber
1 Sliced small zucchini
2 Sliced tomatoes
1/2 Cup mung bean sprouts, chopped
1/4 Cup sunflower sprouts or seeds
1 Teaspoon herbs (thyme, basil, oregano)
2 Tablespoons cold pressed oil
2 Tablespoons apple cider vinegar (or
        lemon juice)
1 Cup cottage cheese

Combine all ingredients except cottage cheese. Make a well in center of salad and fill with cottage cheese. Serves 6.

• • •

MOLDED GARDEN CHEESE SALAD

1 Envelope unflavored gelatin
1/2 Cup cold water (distilled)
16 Ounces low-fat cottage cheese
1/2 Cup shredded carrot
1/3 Cup thinly sliced zucchini, quartered
1/4 Cup finely chopped green onion
1/4 Cup thinly sliced radishes
1/2 Teaspoon garlic salt
Lettuce leaves

In small saucepan, sprinkle gelatin over water to soften; stir over low heat until gelatin dissolves. Cool. In medium bowl, combine remaining ingredients except lettuce. Mix well. Stir in gelatin. Turn into lightly oiled 3-cup mold. Chill until firm. Unmold onto lettuce. Refrigerate leftovers.

AVOCADO LUNCHEON SALAD

1 Large orange
2 Avocados
Fresh lime or lemon juice
Sea salt
Salad greens
1 Cup low-fat cottage cheese

Pare and section orange. Chill. Cut each avocado into halves. Sprinkle with juice and salt. Arrange ingredients attractively on greens. Serve homemade mayonnaise or other dressing separately, if desired. Serves 4.

● ● ●

CABBAGE AND APPLE SLAW

1 Pound head of cabbage
1/2 Cup homemade mayonnaise
3 Tablespoons lemon juice
1 Tablespoon honey
1/2 Teaspoon sea salt
1/4 Teaspoon allspice, ground
1/8 Teaspoon Tabasco sauce
2 Apples, thinly sliced
1/2 Cup chopped pecans

Shred cabbage into a large bowl. Combine mayonnaise, lemon juice, honey, salt, allspice, and Tabasco sauce in a small bowl; mix well. Pour over cabbage and mix. Cover; chill for 1 hour. Just before serving, coat apple slices with a little lemon juice to prevent them from turning dark and arrange around edge of salad. Sprinkle pecans in center. Serves 4.

ROAST SALAD

Left over roast
1 Large apple
1 Large to medium onion
1 Boiled egg
1 Fresh tomato
2 Stalks fresh celery

Chop roast, apple, onion, egg, tomatoes, and celery. Mix together. Add homemade mayonnaise, to taste. Serve on whole wheat bread.

● ● ●

CHICKEN SALAD

1 Chicken (boiled)
1 Boiled egg
2 Apples
1 Onion
2 Fresh Tomatoes
3 Stalks celery
1/2 Cup chopped pecans
1 Cup seedless grapes (halved)

Bone and chop chicken (without skin). Chop other ingredients and mix all together. Add homemade mayonnaise to taste. Mix in 1 tablespoon lemon juice. Sprinkle with pecans. Serve on lettuce leaves, make sandwiches, or stuff tomatoes.

● ● ●

HINT: Always skin chicken before cooking. Most of the fat is in the skin.

HOT CHICKEN SALAD

3/4 Cup diced cooked chicken (without skin)
1/2 Cup thinly sliced celery
1 Tablespoon chopped pimento
1/4 Teaspoon grated onion
2 Avocados
Fresh lime or lemon juice
Sea salt
1 Egg white
Cayenne
Homemade mayonnaise

Combine chicken, celery, pimento, onion, and 1 tablespoon mayonnaise. Cut avocado into halves. Sprinkle with lime/lemon juice and salt. Place cut side up in shallow baking pan. Heat with chicken mixture. Beat egg white until stiff and fold in 1/4 cup mayonnaise. Cover half shells with this mixture and sprinkle with cayenne. Pour warm water about 1/4 inch deep in bottom of pan. Bake in slow oven (300 degrees) for 20 minutes. Serve at once. Serves 4.

● ● ●

GOURMET POTATO SALAD

1 Avocado
2 Tsp. sea salt
1 Cup homemade
  mayonnaise
1/2 Cup sliced
  radishes

4 Cups diced cold
  cooked new potatoes
2 Tablespoons green
  onion

Cut avocado into cubes. Combine with all remaining ingredients, mixing gently. Chill and serve.

95

ORANGE SALAD

Assorted salad greens
Orange slices
Onion slices

Arrange attractively and dribble with orange juice or French
Dressing.

● ● ●

PRUNE SALAD

Cut up navel oranges, bananas, and pitted prunes that have
been soaked to plump them. Top with cottage cheese or
yogurt. Refrigerate leftovers.

● ● ●

CHEESE AND RED BEAN SALAD

16 Oz. low-fat cottage cheese	15 Oz. kidney beans, cooked and drained
1/2 Cup chopped green pepper	1/2 Cup sliced pimento stuffed olives
1/2 Cup chopped onion	1/2 Teaspoon sea salt
1/4 Teaspoon cayenne	Lettuce leaves

In large bowl, combine all ingredients except lettuce, mix
well. Chill. Serve on lettuce. Refrigerate leftovers.

Mexican Foods

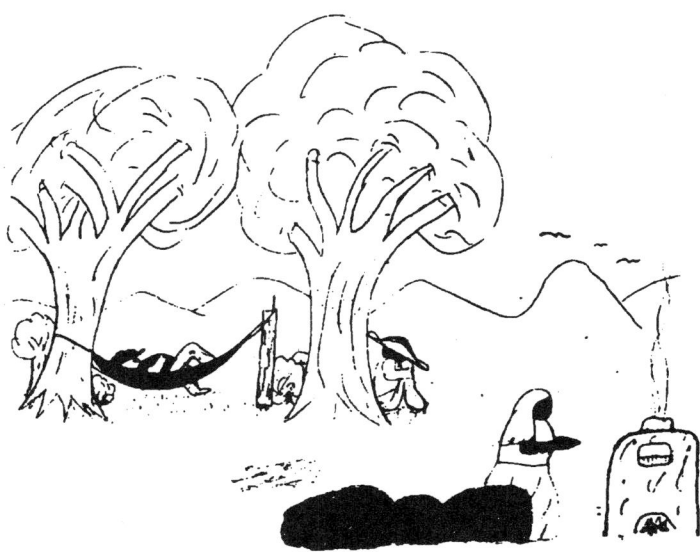

STEAK

Very lean thick steaks
Homemade tomato sauce
Garlic (optional)
Almonds
Raisins

Slice holes in steak and stuff with almonds and raisins. Place steak in a Brown and Serve Bag. Pour tomato sauce with a little garlic added over the steak. Bake at 375 degrees. Just before it is well done remove the steak and slice it into 1/2 inch slices. Return to sauce and cook until tender.

● ● ●

"BROWN IN" FISH

Place filet of white flesh fish in Brown In Bag. Pour 1 cup fresh or frozen orange juice over the fish and bake in 350 degree oven until done. About 20 minutes depending on size of filet.

● ● ●

ORANGE CHICKEN

Place chicken (without skin) in a Brown In Bag and pour on 1 cup fresh or frozen orange juice. Bake at 350 degrees. You may cook it alone or add your favorite seasoning; Rosemary, garlic, or both.

ALMOND CHICKEN

Make slits in chicken (without skin) and insert almonds and raisins. Place in Brown In Bag and pour over chicken 1 cup of orange juice. Add prunes around the chicken. Cook in 350 degrees oven until brown.

● ● ●
TACO SALAD

2 Pounds ground beef
1 Medium head of lettuce
3 Tomatoes
1 Large onion
1 8 oz. Package non fat cottage cheese
Homemade corn chips or tortillas

Brown beef and drain off excess fat. Chop lettuce, tomatoes, onion and mix with beef. Stir in cottage cheese. Serve over homemade corn chips or tortillas that have been broken into small pieces. Pour salsa on top.

● ● ●
SALSA

2 Medium tomatoes, diced
1 Medium onion, diced
1/4 Cup parsley, chopped
1 Clove garlic, minced
1/2 Teaspoon sea salt
1/8 Teaspoon cayenne
1/8 Teaspoon ground cumin

Combine tomatoes, onion, parsley, garlic, sea salt, cayenne, and cumin in a small bowl. Refrigerate 1 hour or until well chilled. Makes 3 cups. Serve with any Mexican dish.

CHILI CORN CHIP

1 Cup yellow cornmeal
1/3 Cup whole wheat flour
3/4 Teaspoon sea salt
1/4 Teaspoon baking soda
1/8 Teaspoon cayenne pepper
3/4 Teaspoon chili powder
1/2 Cup buttermilk
3 Tablespoons cold pressed oil
2 Teaspoons coarse salt

Toast 1/2 cup cornmeal in a shallow pan in a 350 degree oven for 15 minutes. Combine with remaining 1/2 cup corn meal, flour, salt, baking soda, cayenne and chili powder in a bowl. Combine buttermilk and oil in a small bowl. Stir into cornmeal mixture until dough forms a ball. Knead on wax paper for about 5 minutes. Divide dough in half. Roll each to make a 12-inch square. Sprinkle with coarse salt; roll lightly with rolling pin to press in salt. Cut into 1-inch squares with knife or pizza cutter. Transfer to lightly greased cookie sheet. Bake at 350 degrees for 15 minutes. Makes 1/2 pound.

● ● ●

HAMBURGER SAUCE

3 Small onions, chopped
1 Lb. very lean ground beef
1 1/2 Cups homemade tomato sauce
2 Teaspoons chili powder
2 Teaspoons sea salt.

Brown onions and ground beef in a skillet for a few minutes stirring with a fork to break meat into bits. Add remaining ingredients and simmer for 45 minutes. **NOTE:** This sauce is excellent over spaghetti, rice or potatoes.

MEXICAN STYLE STEAK

1 Lb. lean round steak
1/2 Teaspoon sea salt
1 Teaspoon chili powder
1/2 Cup flour
4 Tablespoons cold pressed oil
1/2 Clove of garlic, minced
1 Onion, chopped fine (medium size)
1 Cup tomatoes

Mix salt, chili powder and flour. Beat all into steak. Fry garlic and onion in oil until tender, add steak and brown on both sides. Add tomatoes and enough water (distilled) to cover. Cover and simmer 45 minutes or until meat is tender. Serves 4.

● ● ●

MEXICAN MEAT PIE

3 Cups cooked rice
1 Cup homemade tomato sauce
1/2 Cup sliced stuffed olives
        (from health food store - bottled with sea salt)
1/2 Teaspoon sea salt
2 Teaspoons chili powder
2 Cups finely chopped cooked meat
1 Cup meat broth
Biscuit dough

Combine rice, tomatoes, olives, seasonings, cooked meat and broth. Pour into well greased casserole or baking dish and bake in moderate oven at 350 degrees for about 30 minutes. Cut small biscuits from biscuit dough, place on top of casserole dish, return to oven and bake at 400 degrees until biscuits are done, about 10 minutes. Serve while hot. Serves 6.

FISH WITH CHILI SAUCE

2 Tablespoons cold pressed oil
1 Onion, chopped
1 Green pepper, chopped
1 Clove garlic, minced
2 Tablespoons flour
1/2 Teaspoon sea salt
1 Tablespoon chili powder
1 Cup tomatoes
1 Cup meat stock or distilled water

Saute onion, green pepper, garlic in oil, add flour, salt, chili powder; stir until smooth; add tomatoes and other liquids; simmer until thick. ●Choose fish suitable for baking, either fillets or whole fish. Place in baking dish and top with rings of green peppers and onions, then cover with the above sauce. Bake in hot oven 400 degrees about ten minutes per pound of fish.

MEXICAN RICE

2 Tablespoons cold pressed oil
1 Cup uncooked rice
1 Cup tomatoes
1 Small onion, minced
1/2 Green pepper, chopped
2 Teaspoons chili powder
2 Cups water (distilled)

Wash rice well; dry; brown raw rice in hot oil, add onion, green pepper, sea salt, chili powder, tomatoes. Mix well; add just enough water to cover. Cover with lid; allow to simmer until rice is tender, about 30 minutes. Remove lid to allow mixture to dry out. Do not stir after cooking starts. Serves 6. ●For an unusual flavor touch from Old Mexico, serve with sliced bananas around rim of serving dish.

MEXICAN STYLE EGGPLANT

3 Tablespoons cold pressed oil
4 Small onions, sliced thin
2 Green peppers, sliced thin
1 Medium eggplant, cubed and peeled
4 Small tomatoes, sliced thin
2 Teaspoons sea salt
2 Teaspoons chili powder

Heat fat, cook onions and peppers until tender; add eggplant, tomatoes. Season with sea salt and chili powder. Cover, simmer 20 minutes over slow fire.

Fine meat substitute.

● ● ●

TORTILLAS
American Style

3 Tablespoons cold pressed oil
1 Teaspoon sea salt
2 Cups flour
3/4 Cup water (distilled)

Sift dry ingredients into mixing bowl; cut in oil, add water to make dough. Roll very thin, on lightly floured board, cut into cakes 5" in diameter. Bake on lightly greased griddle; turn frequently to brown evenly. Press with pancake turner to keep cakes flat. Drain on absorbent paper. Makes 1 dozen.

TORTILLAS

1 Cup cornmeal
1 Cup boiling water (distilled)
1 Teaspoon sea salt
2 Teaspoons cold pressed oil

Stir boiling water into cornmeal. Add salt, oil and mix well. Pat into very thin cakes, bake on greased griddle; turn as they brown. Makes about 1 dozen.

Vegetables

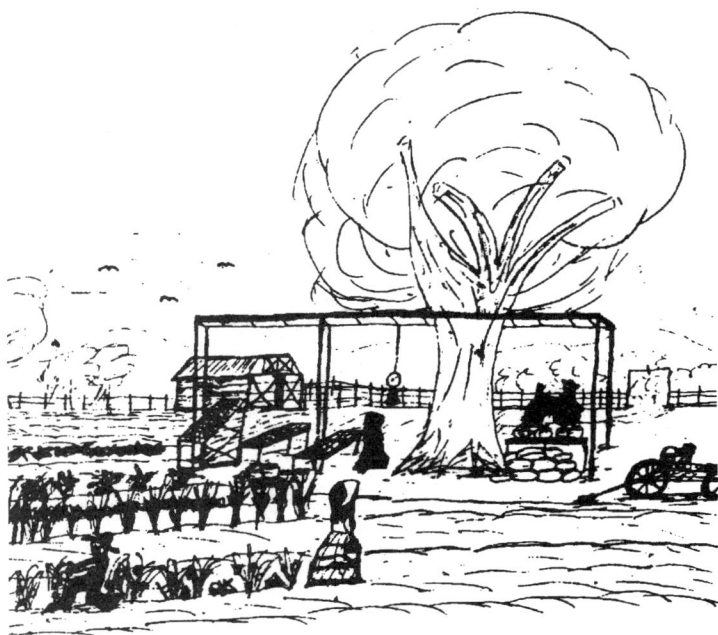

VEGETABLES

The best and most nutritious way to cook vegetables is to steam them. All health food stores stock the stainless steel collapsible steamers that fit into any size pan. Vegetables are delicious steamed over chicken (without skin) broth. If you must have seasoning on vegetables, wait until they are cooked.

Vegit is an all vegetable seasoning to use in place of salt. Spike is an herb seasoning with a trace of sea salt. Kelp powder gives vegetables a new and tasty flavor. Experiment to develop new tastes.

I have included as many unusual vegetable dishes as I could find. I have included salt and butter, but it would be well to try to cut down on these seasonings as much as possible.

A very good seasoning for vegetables is sesame butter. The recipe is included in the Dressings, Sauces, and Butters Chapter.

Sandra experimented with sesame butter and found it unsuitable for sauteing, but very good for seasoning any cooked vegetable dish.

The following is a list of the most nutritious vegetables. They should all be included in your diet either raw, juiced, or steamed. I obtained this information from a February, 1979 Organic Gardening article.

After you read and realize all the valuable nutrients in these foods, nutrients so essential to full optimum health, I am sure you will come to the same conclusion I have. What a shame to boil all these valuable elements out and pour them down the drain!

CARROTS

Carrots are first among all the vegetables for Vitamin A content. One old wives tale that carrots are good for your eyesight is one that happens to be true. Carrots also have generous amounts of potassium and calcium.

SWEET POTATOES

Sweet potatoes rank only second to carrots, for Vitamin A content. It is also high in thiamine.

CAULIFLOWER

Cauliflower is another high source of Vitamin C. It also contains thiamine, iron, and riboflavin.

BROCCOLI

Broccoli is probably the most nutritious of all vegetables and should become a favorite of all cancer patients, since it has a high potency of Vitamin A and Vitamin C. It is also very high in iron, calcium, riboflavin (Vitamin B), potassium, thiamine, and niacin.

SPINACH

Another great source of Vitamin A. As for minerals, spinach is high in iron, potassium, and calcium. It also has a high content of the Vitamin B riboflavin.

BRUSSELS SPROUTS

Brussels sprouts are important to cancer patients because they are very high in Vitamin C. The B Vitamin riboflavin is very high also. As for minerals, brussels sprouts contain iron, potassium, niacin, thiamine, and calcium.

PEAS

Peas are high in all the B Vitamins and Vitamin C; also thiamine, niacin, riboflavin, and iron.

ARTICHOKES

Artichokes have plentiful amounts of calcium, niacin, iron, and especially potassium.

STEAMING

Steaming is the second best method to prepare vegetables. Of course, raw takes first place. If you wish to eat your vegetables cooked, steaming retains all the flavor and color. You also lose much less nutrients than you do in boiling. Boiling destroys 90 to 95 percent of all the vitamins and minerals. What few are left are mostly in the water and usually go down the kitchen sink. If you steam vegetables ahead of time, be sure to remove them from the steamer and run cold water over them to stop the cooking process. To reheat, place over boiling water two or three minutes. Never simmer vegetables for a long time as it does the same damage to them as boiling.

Here are some tested times for steaming vegetables:

VEGETABLE	MINUTES
Asparagus	7 - 10
Carrots	7 - 10
Cabbage	8 - 9
Broccoli	10 - 12
Cauliflower	14
Spinach	2 - 4
String beans	10 - 12
Peas	6 - 7
Potatoes	1 hour
New small potatoes	12 - 15

VEGETABLE	MINUTES
Sweet potatoes	34 - 40
Raisins	3
Mushrooms	7
Squash	5

• • •

HINTS FOR STEAMED VEGETABLES

To dress up plain steamed vegetables try some of these toppers:

- Add sauteed mushrooms, chopped walnuts, or toasted sesame seed.
- Toss lightly with sesame seed butter seasoned with Vegit.
- Dash a pinch of most any herb on top before steaming.
- Add a few sprouts to make any vegetable more interesting.
- Top with sauteed onions.
- Sliced raw radishes give a crunchy, nutty flavor.
- Make croutons out of whole wheat bread and season with Kelp or Vegit.
- Trim with strips of fresh pimento or sprig of fresh mint.
- Parsley is always a pretty decoration but be sure to eat it.
- Slivered almonds are a mainstay to dress up green beans.

VEGETABLE COMBINATIONS

Steam vegetables separately, then mix together for added mealtime variety.
(See Steaming Guide)

Cauliflower and green peas

Onions and green peas

Carrot slices and green lima beans

Tomatoes and zucchini

Mushrooms and green peas

Green lima beans in acorn squash

Diced carrots in nest of French style green beans

Celery and mushrooms

Carrots and green peas

Okra and tomatoes

Celery and carrots

Brussels sprouts and celery

Tomatoes, onion, and summer squash

Corn and green lima beans

Red cabbage and green cabbage

Brussels sprouts and carrot slices

Green peas and corn

EGGPLANT - ZUCCHINI DISH

1 Medium eggplant (about 1 1/2 pounds)
2 Small zucchini
1 Cup finely chopped green pepper
1 Medium onion, finely chopped (about 1/2 cup)
4 Medium tomatoes, peeled and quartered
1/4 cup cold pressed oil
2 Teaspoons sea salt

Prepare 5 cups cubed pared eggplant. Prepare 2 cups - 1/2 inch sliced zucchini. Cook and stir in all ingredients until heated through. Cover; cook over medium heat, stirring occasionally, about 10 minutes or until vegetables are crisp-tender. 6 to 8 servings.

● ● ●

TOMATOED CORN

4 Ears fresh corn or 1 package (10 ounces)   frozen whole kernel corn
1/4 Cup raw butter
1/4 Cup chopped onion
1/4 Cup chopped green pepper
2 Teaspoons honey
1/2 Teaspoon sea salt
1/4 Teaspoon ground cumin
1 Large tomato

If fresh corn, husk and remove silk; cut enough kernels from ears to measure 2 cups. Cook and stir all ingredients except tomato over medium heat until raw butter is melted. Cover; cook 10 minutes longer. Stir in tomatoes. Cover; cook 5 minutes.

CORN SAUTE

3 Ears fresh corn
3 Tablespoons raw butter
1 Clove garlic, crushed
2 Tablespoons sesame seed
2 Tablespoons chopped green pepper
1/2 Teaspoon sea salt
1/4 Teaspoon basil leaves

Husk corn and remove silk; cut enough kernels from ears to measure 1 1/2 cups. Cook and stir all ingredients over medium heat until raw butter is melted. Cover; cook over low heat 15 minutes or until corn is tender.

For Frozen Corn:
Use 1 package (10 ounces) frozen whole kernel corn and cook, stirring occasionally, 7 minutes or until corn is tender.

● ● ●

FRESH CARROTS IN PINEAPPLE SAUCE

1 1/4 Lbs. fresh carrots
1/4 Cup raw butter, melted
1/4 Cup fresh pineapple juice
1 Teaspoon honey

Heat oven to 375 degrees. Scrape carrots; remove ends. Cut carrots into long strips about 1/4 inch thick. Place in ungreased baking dish.

Stir together raw butter, honey, and pineapple juice. Pour over carrots. Cover, bake 40 minutes or until carrots are tender. Serves 4.

CARROTS WITH CHIVES

1 1/2 Lbs. fresh carrots
1/4 Cup raw butter
1/4 Teaspoon sea salt
1 Tablespoon snipped chives

Steam carrots (see Steaming Guide). Melt raw butter in medium skillet; add carrots. Sprinkle with sea salt and snipped chives. Heat carrots through, turning occasionally to coat with butter.

● ● ●

VEGETABLE MEDLEY

1 Small head green cabbage (about 1 pound)
1 Tablespoon cold pressed oil
1 Cup thin diagonal sliced celery
1 Medium green pepper, cut into thin
    diagonal slices
2/3 Cup chopped onion
1 Teaspoon sea salt

Steam cabbage (See Steaming Guide). Heat cold pressed oil in medium skillet. Add vegetables and stir. Cover, steam 5 minutes or until crisp tender, stirring several times. Add sea salt. If desired, stir in 1 tablespoon soy sauce. Serves 4.

● ● ●

TURNIP WITH PARSLEY AND LEMON

Steam 2 cups turnip sticks (See Steaming Guide). Add 2 teaspoons snipped parsley, 1 tablespoon raw butter, 1 teaspoon finely chopped onion, and 1 teaspoon lemon juice. Toss. Serves 4.

CHINESE ASPARAGUS

Prepare 2 pounds fresh asparagus. Cut each stalk on the diagonal into 1 - inch pieces. In large skillet, heat 1/3 cup raw butter and 1/3 cup water (distilled) to boiling. Add asparagus, 1/2 teaspoon sea salt. Cover; cook over low heat until asparagus is crisp-tender. (Do not overcook.)

With frozen asparagus - use 2 packages (10 ounce each) frozen asparagus cuts; melt the raw butter with sea salt and omit the 1/3 cup water.

● ● ●

EASTERN SPINACH

Wash and pat dry 1 pound fresh spinach. Remove stems and cut into 1 - inch pieces. Tear leaves into bite-size pieces. Heat 2 tablespoons cold pressed oil and 1 table-spoon Tamari soy sauce in skillet; add spinach, stems and leaves. Cover-cook 1 minute or until just wilted. Uncover and toss till spinach is tender-crisp and well coated, about 2 minutes. Serves 4.

● ● ●

NEW POTATOES AND PARSLEY

Scrub 1 1/2 lbs. tiny new potatoes. Steam (See Steaming Guide). Meanwhile, melt 1/4 cup raw butter in saucepan; stir in 1/4 cup snipped parsley and 1 tablespoon lemon juice. Pour over hot potatoes. Serves 4 to 6.

NEW POTATOES WITH CREAMED PEAS

1 1/2 Lbs. (about 15) tiny new potatoes
1 to 1 1/2 cups fresh peas (1 to 1/ 1/2
    lbs. in shell)
3 Tablespoons sliced green onion
4 Teaspoons raw butter
4 Teaspoons whole wheat flour
1 Cup powdered milk

Scrub potatoes; pare off narrow strip of peel around center of each. Steam potatoes, peas and onion. (See Steaming Guide). Make a sauce of raw butter, whole wheat flour, and milk. Combine vegetables and sauce. Serves 4 to 6.

● ● ●

FRESH PEAS

2 Lbs. fresh unshelled peas
3 to 6 lettuce leaves
1/3 Cup sliced green onion
1 Teaspoon honey
1/2 Teaspoon sea salt
Dash dried thyme, crushed
3 Tablespoons raw butter

Shell peas. Cover bottom of skillet with lettuce; top with peas and onion. Pour on honey and sprinkle with seasoning; add raw butter. Cover tightly and cook over low heat 10 to 15 minutes or till peas are done. Serves 4.

● ● ●

CAULIFLOWER AND PEAS

2 Tablespoons cold pressed oil
2 Cups small fresh cauliflowerettes
2 10-ounce packages frozen peas
1/2 Teaspoon sea salt
2 Tablespoons chopped fresh pimento

Heat oil in skillet. Add cauliflowerettes and cook covered over low heat 10 to 12 minutes stirring occasionally. Add peas and pimento, sea salt. Cover and cook 10 minutes longer, separating peas with fork if necessary. Makes 8 servings.

● ● ●

SQUASH WITH DILL WEED

Slice 1 lb. yellow summer squash crosswise 1/4 inch thick. Melt 2 tablespoons raw butter in skillet; add squash, 1 tablespoon snipped parsley, 1/4 teaspoon dried dill weed, dash onion powder and 1/4 teaspoon sea salt. Cover skillet and cook over low heat 8 to 10 minutes or till tender. Stir occasionally. Serves 4 to 6.

● ● ●

JAPANESE CELERY

Slice 8 large outside stalks on the bias. Steam over boiling water till crisp-tender. Drain. Cook 1 cup sliced fresh mushrooms in 3 tablespoons raw butter till tender; add celery and 1/4 cup almond halves. Toss lightly till hot. Makes 6 servings.

MUSHROOM SAUTE

1 PINT (about 1/2 lb.) fresh mushrooms. Slice through cap and stem. Melt 3 tablespoons raw butter in skillet; add fresh mushrooms. Sprinkle with 2 teaspoons whole wheat flour; toss to coat. Cover; cook over low heat till tender 8 to 10 minutes, turning occasionally. Serve as a vegetable or as meat accompaniment.

• • •

BROILED TOMATOES

2 - 3 Large firm tomatoes
1/4 Cup whole wheat crumbs
1 Tablespoon raw butter
1 Teaspoon honey

Slice tomatoes into 3/4 to 1-inch slices. Pour honey over tomatoes before placing in buttered pan, sprinkle crumbs on slices and dot with raw butter. Broil on first shelf from heat until crusty brown, lower if necessary to cook. Broiling time takes about 7 minutes.

• • •

BRUSSELS SPROUTS AND FIXINGS

Sprinkle steamed sprouts lightly with ground nutmeg, crushed sage, or caraway.

Add water chestnuts to sprouts for added crispness.

Toss cooked sprouts with sesame butter and warm whole wheat croutons.

BRUSSELS SPROUTS POLONAISE

2 Lbs. Brussels sprouts
1/4 Cup raw butter
1/4 Cup fine dry whole wheat bread crumbs
1 Hard cooked egg yolk, sieved
2 Tablespoons snipped parsley

Cut large sprouts in half. Steam till tender. (See Steaming Guide). Drain. Heat raw butter in small saucepan till it begins to brown; add whole wheat bread crumbs, egg yolk, and parsley. Spoon over sprouts; toss lightly. Serves 6 to 8.

● ● ●

GREEN BEANS AND ALMONDS

2 Lbs. fresh or frozen green beans
1 Cup almonds, in slivers
2 Tablespoons butter
Sea salt to taste

If using fresh beans, choose bright green, crisp, small green beans. Snap off ends or slice beans on the bias. Steam beans according to instructions in "Steaming", "Tested Times for Steaming Vegetables" and "Tested Times for Steaming Frozen Vegetables".

You can prepare the beans earlier by running cold water over them to stop the cooking. You will preserve the nice green color. Set aside until ready to use. Add raw almonds to the green beans, and serve hot.

SUNNY CARROTS

5 Medium carrots
1 Tablespoon honey
1 Teaspoon cornstarch
1/4 Teaspoon sea salt
1/4 Teaspoon ground ginger
1/4 Cup fresh orange juice
2 Tablespoons raw butter

Cut carrots lengthwise into 1-inch chunks. Cook, covered in boiling sea salted water till tender, about 20 minutes. Drain. Meanwhile, combine honey, cornstarch, sea salt and ground ginger in a small saucepan. Add fresh orange juice; cook stirring constantly, till mixture thickens and bubbles. Boil 1 minute. Stir in raw butter. Pour over hot carrots, tossing to coat evenly. Serves 4.

● ● ●

HERBED CARROTS

In heavy saucepan, combine 2 tablespoons raw butter, 1/4 cup water (distilled), 1 tablespoon honey and 1/4 teaspoon dried tarragon, crushed. Add 4 cups quartered carrots (about 1 lb.). Cover lightly; cook over low heat 25 minutes. Sprinkle with 1 teaspoon snipped parsley. Serves 6.

● ● ●

BASIL CARROTS

In medium skillet, melt 2 tablespoons raw butter. Add 6 carrots, thinly diced on the bias. Sprinkle 1/4 teaspoon sea salt and 1/4 teaspoon dried basil, crushed. Cover, simmer 10 to 12 minutes or till tender. Serves 6.

MINTED CARROTS

Combine 2 tablespoons raw butter, 1 tablespoon honey and 2 teaspoons chopped fresh mint. Heat to melt raw butter. Cut 5 to 6 carrots in strips, cooked and drained. Simmer till glazed about 8 minutes. Serves 4 to 5.

● ● ●

HERB GREEN BEANS

Cook 1 lb. fresh green beans, cut in 1-inch lengths; cover in small amount boiling sea salted water 10 minutes; drain. Stir in 2 tablespoons raw butter, 1/2 cup chopped onion, 1/4 cup chopped celery, 1 clove garlic, minced, 1/4 teaspoon dried rosemary, crushed, and 1/4 teaspoon dried basil, crushed. Cover; cook 10 minutes over low heat till tender. Season to taste with sea salt. Serves 6 to 8.

● ● ●

STEAMED TOMATOES AND OKRA

Steam 1 1/2 cups fresh okra in 1/2 inch slices. (See Steaming Guide). Cook 1/2 cup chopped onion and 1/2 cup chopped green pepper in 2 tablespoons cold pressed oil till tender but not brown; blend in 1 tablespoon honey, 1 teaspoon whole wheat flour, 3/4 teaspoon sea salt. Add 3 tomatoes quartered and okra. Serves 4.

● ● ●

PIMENTO SQUASH

Steam (See Steaming Guide) small summer squash, (less than 3 inches long) till tender. Split lengthwise and brush cut surface with melted raw butter. Season with sea salt. Sprinkle with snipped parsley and chopped fresh pimento.

GLAZED STEAMED CARROTS

12 - 15 Whole, young, thin carrots, peeled
2 Tablespoons honey
2 Tablespoons butter

Steam carrots (See Steaming) as follows: Bring 4 cups water (distilled) to boil in saucepan. Place steamer in before adding carrots; put lid on, boil until steam appears. Reduce heat to medium - high; steam about 15 minutes. If you wish, taste the carrots to see that they are firm, but done as you like them. Remove carrots to very small skillet heated with butter and honey. Glaze by rolling the carrots around in mixture on medium heat until glazed, about 4 - 5 minutes.

● ● ●

RICED POTATOES

Cooking time: 25 minutes.

Boil Idaho potatoes, peeled and cut in half, in sea salted water to cover in saucepan. Bring to boil on high heat, reduce to medium, place lid on, cook on low until soft. Drain off water and dry potatoes. Put potatoes, a few at a time, through ricer, being careful not to crush potatoes as you rice them. Sprinkle with sea salt and a lump of sesame butter. Serve at once.

WAX BEANS AND ALMONDS

1 Lb. fresh wax beans
1/2 Cup water (distilled)
2 Tablespoons raw butter
3/4 Teaspoon sea salt
3 Tablespoons toasted slivered almonds

Wash beans and remove ends. Leave beans whole, cut French-style into lengthwise strips or crosswise into 1-inch pieces. Cook beans, water, butter, salt over medium heat until butter is melted. Stir, cover, simmer for 20 to 25 minutes. Stir in almonds.

● ● ●

GARDEN VEGETABLE BAKE

10 Ounces mixed vegetables, cooked and
   drained
1 Cup low-fat cottage cheese
2 Eggs, beaten
1/4 Cup soft whole wheat bread crumbs
1 Tablespoon minced onion
2 Teaspoons lemon juice
1/2 to 1 Teaspoon sea salt
1/4 Teaspoon marjoram leaves

Preheat oven to 350 degrees. In medium bowl, combine ingredients; mix well. Turn into well-greased 1 quart baking dish. Bake 25 minutes. Refrigerate leftovers.

STUFFED BAKED POTATOES

4 Large baked potatoes
1 Cup low-fat cottage cheese
2 Tablespoons chopped chives
1 1/2 Teaspoons sea salt
1/8 Teaspoon cayenne
3 Tablespoons raw butter
2 to 4 Tablespoons low-fat milk
Pimento strips

Preheat over to 400 degrees. Cut potatoes in half and scoop out pulp, reserve shells. In large mixer bowl, combine potato, cheese, chives, salt, cayenne, and butter; beat until fluffy, adding enough milk for desired consistency. Fill shells; place on baking sheet. Bake 12 to 15 minutes or until hot. Refrigerate leftovers.

● ● ●

STUFFED PEPPERS

Cut stem ends out of 3 green peppers and remove seeds. Steam 10 minutes. For stuffing combine:

1 Cup diced celery
2 Tablespoons chopped onion
1 1/2 Cups cooked brown rice

Season with 1 teaspoon Spike or Vegit. Bake in dish that has been greased with cold pressed oil for 30 minutes. Fresh corn may be used instead of rice.

SPINACH LOAF

1 Tablespoon cold pressed oil
1 Chopped onion
1 Cup uncooked cracked wheat
2 Cups water (distilled)
1/2 Teaspoon sea salt
2 Cups cooked spinach
1 Cup walnuts
2 Eggs
1 1/2 Teaspoons sea salt

Saute onion and wheat in oil (not over 240 degrees) till onion is transparent. Add water and 1/2 teaspoon salt. Bring to a boil, cover, then lower heat and simmer 15 minutes or until all water is absorbed. Place spinach, walnuts and eggs in blender and blend at high speed until pureed. Pour mixture into large bowl and stir in cracked wheat and 1 1/2 teaspoons salt. Spread in 9x5x3 inch oiled loaf pan. Bake at 350 degrees for 55 minutes. Let stand 5 to 10 minutes before removing from pan.

● ● ●

STUFFED SQUASH

2 Cups mashed squash
1 Teaspoon cold pressed oil
2 Tablespoons honey

Beat ingredients together. Shape into cups and fill with steamed green peas. Serves 3.

ZUCCHINI MEXICAN STYLE

Wash and stem about 8 or 9 medium sized zucchini, cut in thin rounds. Season with sea salt and paprika. Heat 4 tablespoons olive oil in heavy skillet, add zucchini; and cook covered for 15 minutes, watching and stirring frequently to avoid its sticking. Add 1 large onion, finely chopped and 3 medium tomatoes (juice and all), also 3 green chilies, finely chopped. Simmer, covered, for another 15 minutes. Near time to serve, add 1/2 cup low-fat milk and about 1/2 cup raw unprocessed cheese, grated. Mix well, place in 1 1/2 quart casserole and bake another 15 minutes or until cheese melts.

• • •

DIRTY RICE

Cook as directed:
2 Cups raw brown rice

Saute in oil:
1 Large onion, chopped
4 Stalks celery, diced
1 Clove garlic, chopped

Dice:
12 Chicken giblets, cooked
1 Bunch green onions

Mix the cooked rice with all ingredients. Heat thoroughly and season with sea salt to your taste. This is good with chicken.

BAKED BEANS WITH ORANGE JUICE

1 Lb. dried white beans
1 Cup tomato sauce
1/2 Cup honey
1/4 Cup frozen concentrated undiluted orange juice
Water (distilled)
2 Tablespoons Tamari soy sauce
1/3 Cup chopped onion
1 Teaspoon sea salt

Soak beans covered with water overnight. Drain and place in large kettle with 6 cups water. Simmer 1 1/2 hours or until tender. Pour into 1 1/2 quart casserole. Add 1/2 cup more water and remaining ingredients; mix. Cover and bake at 325 degrees for 4 hours, stirring occasionally. Serve with Orange Salad and Orange French Dressing.

● ● ●

STUFFED SWEET POTATOES

3 Large sweet potatoes, cooked in jackets
1/4 Cup raisins
1/2 Cup walnuts
1/2 Cup sesame seeds
1 Cup fresh cranberries

Put cranberries, walnuts, sesame seeds and raisins through food chopper. Cut potatoes in half lengthwise, and spoon out centers and mash. Mix all ingredients together and fill potatoes. Bake at 350 degrees for 30 minutes.

BROWN BEANS
(BRUNA BONOR)

1 Package (1 lb.) brown beans
   (or red kidney beans)
6 Cups water
1 Cinnamon stick
2 Tablespoons unsalted raw butter
1/2 Cup dark molasses (unsulphured)
2 Teaspoons sea salt
2 to 4 Teaspoons apple vinegar
Cornstarch (optional)

Rinse and pick over the beans. Place in 12 quart pan, add water and let soak overnight. Add butter and whole cinnamon sticks, bring to boiling and then lower heat. Cover. Simmer, stirring occasionally for 1 1/2 hours or until beans are almost tender. Add molasses, salt and vinegar and continue cooking, stirring often and adjusting lid to partially cover pan. Cook for 30 minutes longer or until beans are completely tender and sauce is brown and slightly thickened. If you wish, the sauce can be thickened with a little cornstarch mixed with cold water.

PILAF

2 Cups cooked wheat
1/2 Cup chopped celery
1/2 Cup chopped onions
2 Tablespoons butter
2 Cups chicken (without skin) broth

Saute onion and celery in butter. Add cooked wheat and saute briefly. Add broth and simmer until liquid is absorbed. Serve in place of potatoes. ●Also may be used to stuff such vegetables as tomatoes, cabbage, peppers, or squash. Bake covered at 350 degrees for 30 minutes.

STUFFED CABBAGE

6 Large cabbage leaves
1/2 Lb. ground lean beef
1 1/2 Shredded wheat biscuits, crumbled
1 Small onion, grated
1 Egg
1/2 Teaspoon sea salt
1 Medium onion, sliced
2 Large tomatoes sliced
2 Cups tomato juice made in blender
1 Lemon
1/4 Cup honey

Shave off thick part of each cabbage leaf and pour boiling water over them to make them easier to fold. Heat oven to 375 degrees. Combine meat with shredded wheat, grated onion, egg, and salt. Place mound of meat mixture in cup of each leaf. Loosely fold over sides of each leaf and roll up. In bottom of Dutch oven, place a few cabbage leaves. Arrange layer of rolled leaves, with seam side down, and sliced onion in Dutch oven. Place sliced tomatoes on top. Pour on tomato juice and juice of lemon. Add salt. Bring to boil on top of range. Dribble honey on top and bake, covered for 1 hour. Uncover; bake 2 hours. Serve with brown rice.

LETTUCE GAZPACHO

3 Peeled tomatoes
4 Celery stalks
1 Medium cucumber, peeled
Lettuce
1/3 Cup orange juice
Juice of 1 lemon
Blend and serve cold as a first course.

GAZPACHO

Chop fine:
4 Large ripe tomatoes, peeled
1/2 Cucumber, peeled

Add:
1/4 Cup chopped green pepper
Dash of tabasco
4 Tablespoons olive oil
4 Teaspoons apple cider vinegar
1 Cup tomato juice
1/2 Teaspoon sea salt
1 Teaspoon grated onion
1 Teaspoon Spike

Chill overnight. Blend in blender 1 minute at high speed.
Serve cold.

• • •

MARINATED MUSHROOMS

1 Lb. fresh mushrooms
1 Pint distilled water
3/4 Cup lemon juice
1 Tablespoon cold pressed oil
1 Bay leaf
Pinch of thyme

Bring water and lemon juice to a boil. Add mushrooms and
cook 3 minutes.
Add remaining ingredients, stir, salt to taste and chill.

MUSHROOM SAUCE

1/2 Cup sliced mushrooms
2 Tablespoons unsalted raw butter
2 Tablespoons unbleached flour
3/4 Cup chicken (without skin) broth
1/2 Cup non-fat milk

Saute mushrooms in oil. Mix flour and chicken broth and add to mushrooms. Slowly add milk. Serve over vegetables.

Main Dishes

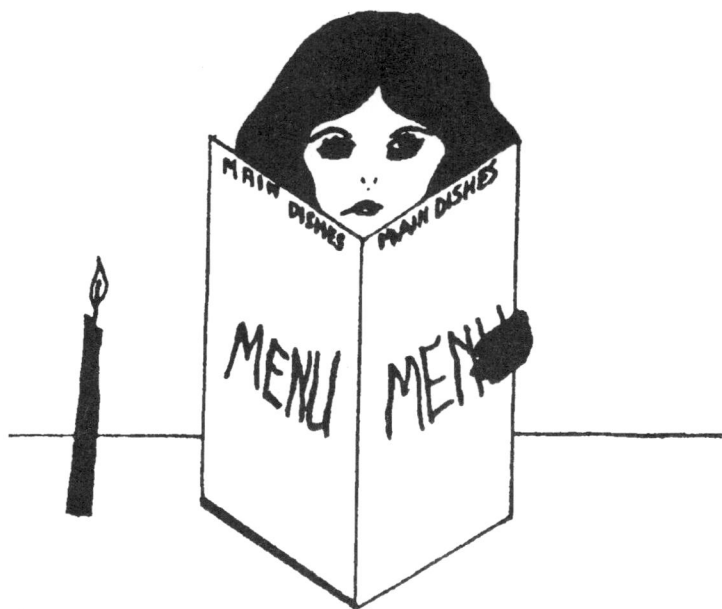

CONCERNING MEAT

There is much controversy among the natural food advocates concerning the eating of meat. I personally do not eat meat, but if you are one of those people who feel you must eat meat, here are a few hints that may make it a little less toxic to your body.

No meat should be eaten from any animals that have been fed or injected with hormones of any kind (as they are definitely carcinogenic), or if they have been fed any chemicals in their food.

If you find meat this pure, only three and one-half ounces are allowed in one day. Alternative doctors recommend that the same animal protein should not be eaten two days in a row. Alternate beef, chicken, and fish. The largest majority of nutritionists recommend no beef whatsoever. The beef recipes in this book are included for those persons who feel the necessity of eating beef. The remaining ingredients in the beef recipes are according to the Laetrile diet.

CASSEROLES

The things I like best about casseroles are that they can be served in the same dish they are cooked in. And they are easily cleaned if before filling them, you grease them slightly with cold pressed oil.

The seasonings and such ingredients as onion or green peppers may be increased, reduced, or left out to suit the family taste. Try many different toppings on casseroles such as toasted wheat germ, sunflower seeds, tomato or green pepper slices arranged in an interesting way. Use your imagination to make all meals more appetizing.

RIPE OLIVE CASSEROLE

3/4 Cup ripe olives
2 Tablespoons cold pressed oil
1/2 Lb. lean ground meat
3/4 Cup chopped onion
1 Cup sliced celery
1 1/2 Teaspoon sea salt
1/4 Teaspoon cayenne
3 Medium tomatoes, chopped
2 Cups wide whole wheat noodles
1 Cup low-fat cottage cheese

Cut olives into small pieces. Heat oil, add meat and cook about 5 minutes, stirring frequently. Stir in onion and celery and cook about 5 minutes longer. Add salt, cayenne, tomatoes, olives, uncooked noodles and cottage cheese. Cover tightly and cook until mixture is boiling. Remove cover and stir lightly but thoroughly. Cover and cook slowly about 20 minutes until noodles are cooked. Serves 4.

CHICKEN PIE

1 4-Lb. chicken (without skin), cut up
1 1/2 Cups hot water (distilled)
3 Celery tops
1 Tablespoon sea salt
1 Bay leaf
1 Large onion
1 Recipe whole wheat biscuits
7 Tablespoons unsalted raw butter
7 Tablespoons unbleached flour
Dash mace
Pinch dried tarragon
1 Teaspoon Spike
1 Cup non-fat milk, thickened with 2
   tablespoons unbleached flour
1 Package frozen peas, hot, cooked

Remove all skin from chicken before cooking. Cook chicken in water and celery tops, salt, onion, and bay leaf. Cut chicken meat into large pieces. Prepare biscuit dough and pat to 1/2 inch thickness, cut into 9 doughnut rings. Make rest of dough into tiny biscuits. Heat oven to 425 degrees. Melt butter in skillet (not over 240 degrees); stir in flour, mace, Spike, tarragon, milk; add 2 cups chicken broth. Cook over medium heat, stirring until thickened. Arrange chicken in 2-quart casserole; pour sauce over all. Arrange biscuit rings around top of pie and brush with a little milk. Bake 25 to 30 minutes or until browned. Cook peas. When pie is done, heap spoonful on top of each biscuit on pie and serve. Cook other biscuits in same oven about 10 minutes. Serves 6.

EAST INDIA CURRY

1 Large chicken (without skin), cut
1 1/2 Cups hot water (distilled)
1 Small onion
2 Celery tops
1/2 Teaspoon sea salt
1/2 Bay leaf
1 Carrot, pared
2 Tablespoons butter
1/2 Cup chopped onion
1/2 Cup chopped celery
1/3 Cup unbleached flour
1 Teaspoon curry powder
1 Teaspoon sea salt
2 3/4 Cups non-fat milk
Snipped parsley

Remove all skin from chicken before cooking. Day before: Simmer chicken in water with onion, celery tops, 1 teaspoon salt, bay leaf, and carrot; covered until tender. Remove; cool slightly, then remove meat from bones; refrigerate until needed. (Meanwhile set kettle of broth in cold water in sink to cool quickly, then refrigerate for later use as soup.) In large kettle, melt butter; add chopped onions and celery. Cook until lightly browned. Then stir in flour, curry and salt. Slowly stir in milk. Cook until thickened stirring constantly. Remove from heat. Then gently add cooked chicken. Quickly cool mixture by setting kettle in cold water in skin, changing cold water as needed. Turn mixture into 1 1/2 quart covered casserole. Refrigerate.

Before serving: bake, covered 1 1/2 hours in 325 degree oven. Just before serving, stir gently with fork. Garnish top with 1 inch border of snipped parsley.

OVEN BEEF STEW

2 Lbs. very lean beef, in 2 inch cubes
1/4 Cup whole wheat flour
3 Tablespoons cold pressed oil
1 Teaspoon sea salt
2 1/2 Cup water (distilled) to tomato juice
12 Small carrots, quartered
6 Medium potatoes, halved
1 Package frozen peas or corn

Start heating oven to 350 degrees. Sprinkle meat with flour, brown in oil in skillet. When browned remove to 3-quart casserole. Stir salt into remaining oil and slowly add water, stirring constantly; then pour over meat. Bake, covered one hour. Add onions, carrots, and potatoes; bake covered, 45 minutes longer. Add peas; bake covered for 15 minutes or until vegetables are tender. Before serving stir stew with fork to bring meat chunks to top. If using corn, omit potatoes. Serves 6.

● ● ●

LIVER AND NOODLES

1/4 Cup cold pressed oil
1 Package frozen peas
1/2 Green pepper, cut into strips
1 Lb. calf liver, cut into 1/2" strips
1/4 Lb. medium whole wheat noodles
1 Cup boiling water (distilled)
1 1/2 Teaspoons sea salt

Saute onions, green pepper and liver in oil 5 minutes, or until tender. Do not heat oil over 240 degrees. Stir in boiling water; peas, salt and uncooked noodles. Cook covered, stirring occasionally to keep from sticking for 10 minutes or until noodles are tender. Serves 4 to 6.

BEEF AND RICE CASSEROLE

1 1/3 Cups cooked brown rice
2 Tablespoons raw butter
1 1/2 Cups diced celery
3 Tablespoons minced onions
1 Lb. ground lean beef
1 Teaspoon Spike
1 Teaspoon sea salt
1 Cup tomatoes blended in blender
1/4 Cup water

Heat oven to 375 degrees. While rice is cooking, saute celery and onions in butter in skillet. Place cooked rice in oiled 1 1/2 quart casserole; top with celery mixture. Season meat with salt and Spike; brown in remaining butter in skillet, then arrange on top of celery. Pour tomatoes on top. Bake 35 minutes. Serves 6.

● ● ●
OKRA TOMATO CASSEROLE

Wash okra. Cut small pods in 1/2 and large ones in 3 or 4 sections. Saute 2 medium onions, finely chopped, in 2 tablespoons olive oil. Slice 6 tomatoes and put a layer of them on the bottom of a buttered 1 1/2 quart casserole. Sprinkle with a pinch of sweet basil. Cover with a layer of okra, season with cayenne pepper, 1/3 of a clove of finely minced garlic, then add a layer of the cooked onion and finely dust with whole wheat bread crumbs. Repeat these layers, topping the whole with a last layer of tomato and a slightly heavier layer of crumbs. Dot with butter and spread a layer of grated unprocessed cheese. Cook covered for one hour at 325 degrees. Uncover and put under broiler for a few seconds to brown the cheese. Replace cover to seal in heat and aroma.

143

MEATLESS CHOP SUEY

2 Tablespoons cold pressed oil
2 Sliced peppers
2 Thinly sliced onions
1 Cup hot water (distilled)
1/2 Teaspoon Vegit
2 Tablespoons arrowroot starch
2 Cups celery, diced
1 Tablespoon Tamari soy sauce
3 Cups mung bean sprouts
Brown rice

Saute peppers, onions, celery, and sprouts for 2 minutes in oil. (Not over 240 degrees.) Cover and cook gently 10 minutes. Combine arrowroot, soy sauce and little water to make a paste. Stir into the vegetable mixture and cook for 2 minutes. Serve over brown rice. Top with a handful of fresh alfalfa sprouts.

● ● ●

HERB CHICKEN

1 Chicken (without skin)
1 Teaspoon marjoram
1 Teaspoon thyme
1 Tablespoon chopped parsley

Wash and dry chicken. Remove skin from chicken. Place in baking dish and sprinkle with marjoram and thyme. Let stand 1 hour and sprinkle with parsley. Dot with marjoram. Bake at 400 degrees for 40 minutes. Makes 4 servings.

CHICKEN a la DON

1 Chicken (without skin), cut in serving pieces
1/2 Cup chopped onion
1/2 Cup chopped celery

Remove skin from chicken. Brown chicken, remove from pan. Saute onion and celery in cold pressed oil. Drain. Return chicken to pan. Cover with 3/4 cup water. Cover pan and let simmer for 1 hour. Excellent with rice.

● ● ●

GARBANZO CHICKEN

1/2 Cup orange juice
1/4 Cup homemade Bar-B-Q sauce
2 Tablespoons sesame seed oil
2 Cups cut up, cooked chicken (without skin)
1 1/2 cups fresh pineapple chunks, soaked
 with 3 tablespoons water
1 Cup garbanzo sprouts
Brown rice

Combine juice, sauce, and oil in saucepan over low heat. Add chicken and pineapple. Heat, but do not boil. Lower heat and add sprouts. Allow sprouts to absorb some heat and juices. Serve on brown rice.

CHICKEN SPAGHETTI

Remove skin from chicken before cooking. Boil chicken in salted water. Remove meat from bones.

Saute:
3 Tablespoons raw butter
1 Diced onion
1 Diced green pepper
1 Cup fresh mushrooms
2 Cups homemade tomato sauce
Pimentos to taste
Sea salt to taste
Garlic salt to taste

Cook whole wheat or zucchini spaghetti in salted water and add to chicken mixture. Heat thoroughly before serving.

● ● ●

LEMON HONEY CHICKEN

1 Chicken (without skin), cut in serving pieces
1/4 Cup honey
2 Tablespoons soy sauce
1 Teaspoon paprika
1 Tablespoon cold pressed oil
1/2 Cup lemon juice
1 Teaspoon grated lemon peel
1/4 Teaspoon nutmeg

Remove skin from chicken. Arrange chicken in baking dish. To make sauce stir together oil, honey, lemon juice, soy sauce, lemon peel, paprika, and nutmeg. Pour sauce over chicken, turning to coat. Bake uncovered in 350 degree oven for 1 hour, or until done. Turn and baste once. Serves 4.

CHICKEN LUAU

Split in two: 2 to 2 1/2 lb. broiler. Remove skin from chicken.

Brush with soy sauce. Broil on broiler rack until medium brown on both sides, then place in large baking dish with cover. Brush chicken generously with softened or melted raw butter.

Along side of each chicken piece place:
   1 Banana, sprinkled lightly with cinnamon and cut in half
   6 - 8 Chunks fresh pineapple
   1/2 Cup sliced fresh mangoes
Cover tightly. Bake in 350 degree oven for thirty minutes. Serves 2.

● ● ●
TEXAS HASH

2 Large onions, sliced
2 Bell peppers, sliced
3 Tablespoons cold pressed oil
3 Stalks celery, finely cut
1 Lb. lean ground beef
2 Cups tomatoes, blended
1 Teaspoon chili powder
1/2 Cup brown rice
1 Teaspoon sea salt

Cook onions, peppers, and celery slowly (not over 240 degrees) in oil until onions are tender. Add meat and saute until it loses its red color. Add tomatoes, rice and salt. Arrange in large casserole. Cover and bake at 375 degrees for 45 minutes.

LASAGNE

Brown and spoon off excess fat: 1 Lb. ground beef

Add:
1 Clove minced garlic
1 Tablespoon parsley flakes
1 Tablespoon basil
1 1/2 Teaspoons sea salt
4 Cups Homemade tomato sauce

Simmer uncovered until sauce is thick, about 45 minutes to 1 hour, stirring occasionally. Cook until tender: 10 Oz. whole wheat lasagne noodles

Drain and rinse in cold water.

Combine:
3 Cups non fat cottage cheese
2 Beaten eggs
2 Teaspoons sea salt
2 Tablespoons parsley flakes

Place half noodles in 9x13 inch baking dish. Spread half of cottage cheese mixture over; add 6 oz. non fat cottage cheese and half the meat sauce. Repeat
layers. Bake at 375 degrees for 30 minutes. Let stand 15 minutes and cut into squares.
Makes 12 servings.

SWEET-N-SOUR BEEF BALLS

Mix together:
1 Lb. very lean ground beef
1 Egg
1 Teaspoon sea salt
1 1/2 Tablespoon onion, chopped fine

Shape into balls and roll in 2 tablespoons whole wheat flour. Saute in 2 tablespoons cold pressed oil, not over 240 degrees.

Add:
1/3 Chicken stock
1 Cup fresh pineapple chunks
3 Green peppers, diced

Simmer over low heat for several minutes.

Make sauce of:
3 Tablespoons cornstarch
2 Teaspoons soy sauce
1/2 Cup apple cider vinegar
1/3 Cup honey
2/3 Cup chicken stock

Stir well, add to meat balls and heat thoroughly. Serve on brown rice or as is.

CHINESE PEPPER STEAK

1 Lb. round steak cut in strips
1/4 Cup cold pressed oil
2 Green peppers, chopped
1/2 Teaspoon honey
1 Cup fresh bean sprouts
4 Green onions, sliced
1 Clove garlic
1/4 Cup soy sauce
1/2 Teaspoon cornstarch
1 1/2 Cups tomatoes

Cook steak until browned in oil, with garlic, green peppers. Then add soy sauce and honey. Simmer for 1 to 4 minutes. Add cornstarch dissolved in 2 tablespoons of cold water. Continue to add bean sprouts, tomatoes (from the blender), and cook this until hot. Top with the sliced green onions.

Serve on brown rice. Makes 4 servings.

• • •

BROILED FISH

Buy fresh white fish and cut into fillets. Lay fish on buttered broiler, skin side down. Sprinkle with dried tarragon, sea salt, and lemon juice. Broil about 3 inches from flame for not more than 7 minutes. Baste with juice in broiler or more lemon juice and broil 5 more minutes. Serve immediately.

FISH POTATO PUFF

1 Cup broiled white fish
1 Cup mashed potato
1 1/2 Tablespoons lemon juice
1 Tablespoon chopped celery
1 Tablespoon parsley
1 Tablespoon minced green pepper
1/2 Teaspoon minced onion
1 Tablespoon raw butter
2 Eggs - separated

Combine fish, potato and lemon juice. Saute celery, parsley, pepper, and onion in butter until tender; add to fish mixture. Add well beaten egg yolks and blend well. Beat egg whites until stiff but not dry and fold into fish. Pile lightly in baking dish with only the bottom oiled. Bake at 350 degrees for 30 to 40 minutes till firm and lightly browned. Do not eat any other recipe with eggs added on the day you eat this. Serves 3.

FISH CASSEROLE

2 Cups cooked fresh white fish
3 Tablespoons unbleached flour
1 1/2 Cups non-fat milk
1/4 Cup diced green pepper
1 Chopped tomato
4 Tablespoons unsalted raw butter
1 Teaspoon sea salt
Few grains cayenne
2 Cups cooked brown rice

Flake fish. Melt 3 tablespoons butter in a saucepan and stir in flour, sea salt, and cayenne. Add milk gradually, cook, stirring constantly till thick. Place rice, fish, tomato, and green pepper in layers in oiled 1 1/2 quart casserole. Begin and end with rice. Pour white sauce over all. Dot with 1 tablespoon butter. Bake at 350 degrees for 20 to 30 minutes.

SOUTHERN STYLE PERCH

1 Small onion
1/4 Green pepper
1/2 Fresh pimento
1/4 Cup soft raw butter
1 Teaspoon sea salt
3/4 Teaspoon chili powder
1/8 Teaspoon thyme
3 Tablespoons dry whole wheat bread crumbs
1 1/2 Lbs. fresh perch fillets

Seed green pepper. Chop onion, green pepper, pimento. Combine onion, green pepper, pimento, raw butter, chili pepper, thyme, and whole wheat bread crumbs; blend well. Place fillets in baking pan; spread raw butter mixture over fillets. Bake 25 - 30 minutes at 425 degrees. Serves 6.

EASTERN RED SNAPPER

1 Large onion
1/2 Green pepper
1 Carrot
3 Stalks celery
2 Pounds fresh red snapper fillet
2 Tablespoons lemon juice
1/2 Teaspoon sea salt
2 Tablespoons olive oil
1 Pound tomatoes (blended in blender)
2 Tablespoons homemade tomato sauce
1/2 Teaspoon sea salt

Chop onion, celery, and carrot. Seed green pepper and chop. Place fish fillets on large plate; sprinkle lemon juice, sea salt, and let stand 30 minutes; place fillets in 9x13 - inch baking pan, discarding excess lemon juice. Heat olive oil in fry pan over medium - high heat; saute onion, green pepper, celery, carrot for 5 minutes stirring with fork. Add blended tomatoes, homemade tomato sauce, sea salt and cover, simmer for 30 minutes. Pour vegetable mixture over fillets; bake 35 minutes at 400 degrees. Serves 6.

SOUTHERN GUMBO

1 Package fresh frozen or fresh okra
3 Tomatoes
1 Medium size onion
1 Green pepper
3 Tablespoons cold pressed oil
Sea salt
1 Teaspoon chili powder

Chop pepper and onion. Add to okra and tomatoes. Season and add a little water (distilled) as needed. Cook slowly in a covered saucepan for about an hour, so that it will be thick.

153

SEAFOOD SPAGHETTI

1 Green pepper, diced
2 Onions, diced
3 Tablespoons raw butter
2 Cups cooked tomatoes
1 1/2 Cup homemade tomato sauce
1 Teaspoon chili powder
1 Small bay leaf
Dash of sea salt
1 Cup cooked fish
8 Ounces spaghetti

Cook green pepper and onions in butter until tender. Add tomatoes, tomato sauce, and seasonings. Cover and simmer 40 to 50 minutes. Cook spaghetti according to directions on package. Add fish to hot sauce, heat through and serve over spaghetti. Serves 4 to 6.

● ● ●

CHICKEN SANDWICHES

8 Slices whole wheat bread toasted with raw butter
3 Cups cubed chicken (skinned and then boiled)
1 1/2 Cups homemade mayonnaise
2/3 Cup chopped celery (finely)
1/2 Cup sliced green onions and tops
1 1/2 Teaspoon curry powder
1 Teaspoon sea salt

Place toast on baking sheet; cover with chicken, sprinkle with sea salt. Cut each sandwich in half. Mix remaining ingredients; spread over chicken to edges of toast. Bake at 375 degrees for 15 minutes. Makes 8 servings.

AVOCADO-CARROT SANDWICH

Combine mashed avocado, grated carrot, and chopped watercress. Spread on any whole grain bread. Add a bunch of sprouts and you have a very tasty treat.

● ● ●

SUPER EGG SALAD SANDWICH

4 Hard-cooked eggs
1/4 Cup homemade mayonnaise
1 Teaspoon mustard
1/2 Teaspoon grated onion
1/2 Teaspoon fresh lime or lemon juice
1/2 Teaspoon sea salt
Dash tabasco sauce
1 Avocado
8 Slices buttered whole wheat bread

Peel and chop eggs. Blend with mayonnaise, mustard, onion, lime juice, salt, and tabasco. Cut avocado into thin slices. Spread egg mixture on half of bread slices, and cover with avocado slices. Top with remaining bread.

Even better with homemade bread!

Wild Rice

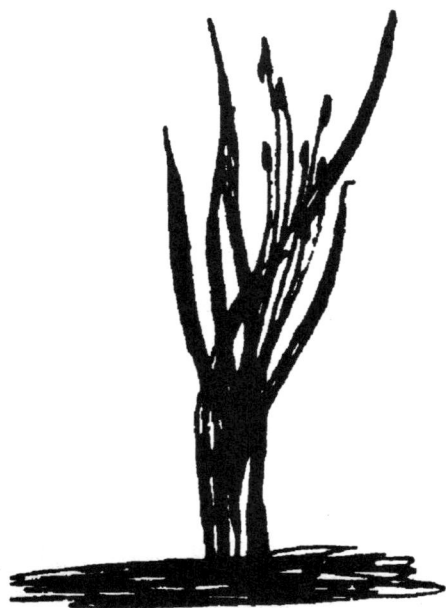

WILD RICE FROM:

KOSBAU BROTHERS, INC.
P.O. Box 599
Grand Rapids, Minnesota 55744

WILD RICE

Wild rice has been an integral part of the diet of the North Central Indians for hundreds of years and today is a popular delicacy throughout the United States.

The distinct nut-like, roasted flavor of wild rice is appealing by itself or when combined with other ingredients the rice adds richness to the dish and enhances the flavor of the other foods.

Wild rice can be precooked, according to one of the methods listed, and refrigerated for a week or more—ready for quick casseroles, salads, or side dishes. No taste is lost in refrigeration.

Wild rice can be "stretched" by substituting some brown rice. Steaming after cooking is very important to increase volume.

Wild rice can be substituted in most recipes that call for white rice; simply allow more cooking time when precooking or 1/2 hour more for oven dishes. The taste can be made milder, if preferred, by changing water one to three times during precooking.

Add wild rice to homemade soups to enhance the flavor.

A generous serving of wild rice contains less than 50 calories. An analysis of one hundred grams (3 1/4 oz.) of uncooked wild rice shows the following:

14.10 Grams protein
339.00 Milligrams phosphorous
.45 Milligrams thiamine
.79 Grams fat
4.20 Milligrams riboflavin
75.00 Grams carbohydrates
7.00 Milligrams sodium
6.20 Milligrams niacin
19.00 Milligrams calcium
220.00 Milligrams potassium

Notice the high potassium content; very important to cancer patients.

Many recipes specify precooked wild rice. Use either the parboiled or baked method unless the recipe states otherwise. Remember that wild rice increases in volume three or more times (1 cup raw makes 3 or more cups cooked rice) after cooking and one cup of raw wild rice equals 6 to 6 1/2 oz.

Wild rice cooks more uniformly if it is graded by size. Cooking time is determined by the amount of dark bran left on the rice during processing. This outer bran layer contains most of the rice's nutrients. Kausbau Brothers, Inc. retain most of this nutritious bran layer.

Prices and information on wild rice may be obtained by writing KOSBAU BROTHERS, INC., P.O. Box 599, Grand Rapids, MN 55744.

PARBOILED WILD RICE

Heat 3 cups water (distilled) and 1 teaspoon sea salt to boiling. Add 1 cup wild rice and lower the temperature to slow simmer. Cover, and cook 30 to 45 minutes until the kernel opens, rice is tender, and the water is absorbed. (Either of the following ways may be used to continue this method.)

A. Drain any excess liquid. Remove cover and fluff with fork. Remove from heat, replace cover, and allow to steep for five minutes.

B. Drain rice in a sieve and place sieve over saucepan containing 1 inch of boiling water. Steam, covered with a folded tea towel, and the lid, for 10 to 15 minutes, or until rice is flaky.

● ● ●

BAKED METHOD

Combine 3 cups water (distilled), 1 cup wild rice, and 1 teaspoon sea salt (beef or chicken bouillon may be added for taste). Place in baking dish, cover, and bake at 325 degrees for 1 1/4 to 1 1/2 hours or until tender. When rice opens, fluff with fork, remove from oven, and leave covered for 5 minutes or more before using.

STUFFED PEPPER N' CHICKEN

1 1/2 Cups wild rice, precooked
6 Medium green peppers
1 Lb. cooked cubed chicken (without skin)
1 Egg
2 Cups tomato sauce mixed with 2 cups water (distilled)
1/2 Teaspoon tabasco sauce
2 Tablespoons Spike
1 Onion, chopped

Mix wild rice, meat, onion, and egg together. Mix soups with rest of ingredients. Pour enough soup mixture into meat mixture to moisten - about 3/4 cup. Stuff this mixture into raw green peppers. Place in deep casserole and pour remaining liquid over the peppers. Bake at 350 degrees for 1 1/2 hours. Serves 6.

● ● ●

ASPARAGUS DELUXE

4 Cups precooked wild rice
2 Cups creamed asparagus
2 Cups chicken (without skin), minced

Mix ingredients together and season with salt and pepper. Let simmer for 10 to 12 minutes. Serves 4 to 6.

CREAMY WILD RICE

2 Cups wild rice, precooked
1 Cup non fat milk
Sea salt, to taste

Simmer 10 minutes. Serve hot with butter or honey. Serves 4.

● ● ●

CONVENIENT COLD CEREAL

Precook (in slightly salted water) wild rice. Drain and keep in refrigerator in air-tight container. Serve cold with low-fat milk or with honey.

If a warm cereal is preferred, simmer wild rice in low-fat milk about 5 minutes and serve with butter or honey. Raisins or dates may be added before simmering if desired.

● ● ●

WILD RICE BISCUITS

1/2 Cup wild rice flour
1 1/2 Cups unbleached four
3 Teaspoons baking powder
1 Teaspoon sea salt
1/4 Cup cold pressed oil
1 Cup non fat milk

Mix all ingredients together and blend well. Spoon heaping tablespoon of batter into greased muffin pan. Bake at 400 degrees for 10 to 12 minutes, until brown. Serve hot. Makes 20 biscuits.

WILD RICE BREAD

2 1/4 Cups lukewarm liquid
    (milk, distilled water or potato water may be used)
4 Teaspoons honey
1 Tablespoon sea salt
4 Tablespoons unsulphured molasses
2 Packages dry yeast
2 Tablespoons cold pressed oil
6 to 6 1/4 cups sifted unbleached flour
1 Cup wild rice flour*

Mix 2 cups liquid, honey, salt, and molasses in a large mixing bowl. Dissolve yeast in 1/4 cup of the warm liquid and stir thoroughly before adding to the rest of the liquid mixture. Add oil. Add flour, 2 cups at a time and blend well after each addition. Knead on lightly floured board until smooth. Place in greased bowl and cover. Let rise till double in bulk. Punch down and knead air out. Divide in half and form into loaves. Place in greased pans and let rise again till doubled in bulk. Bake at 425 degrees for 25 to 30 minutes. Makes 2 loaves.

*100% pure ground wild rice flour may be ordered from Kosbau Bros., Inc.

CASHEW CASSEROLE

1 1/2 Cups wild rice, raw
1 Lb. fresh mushrooms, sliced
1/4 Cup raw butter
1/3 Cup cashews, chopped
Chopped parsley
Sea salt to taste

Rinse wild rice. Place in saucepan and cover with cold water and bring to boil. Drain. Repeat 3 times. The third time add 1 teaspoon salt to the water. Drain well. Saute mushrooms in butter and pour over wild rice; then fold in cashews and mix lightly. Serves 8.

● ● ●

BUTTERMILK WILD RICE PANCAKES

1/4 Cup wild rice flour
2 Eggs
2 Cups buttermilk
2 Tablespoons butter, melted
1 Teaspoon sea salt
2 Cups unbleached flour
2 Tablespoons honey
2 Teaspoons baking powder
1 Teaspoon baking soda

Beat eggs until light and fluffy; stir in buttermilk. Sift together dry ingredients. Gradually add the four to the liquid, beating after each addition to make a smooth and rather thin batter. Stir in melted butter and precooked wild rice. Drop by 1/4 cup onto hot buttered griddle, turning once. Makes 16 - 18 pancakes.

STOVETOP WILD RICE PILAF

1 Cup wild rice, raw
1/4 Cup raw butter
1/4 Cup onion, finely chopped
1/2 Cup sliced mushrooms, sauteed
1 Teaspoon sea salt
1 Cup beef or chicken (without skin) broth
1/3 Cup pimento, chopped
1/4 Cup parsley, chopped

Wash wild rice under hot running water. Drain. In 3 quart skillet, melt butter and add onion, mushrooms, uncooked wild rice and salt. Add broth and 2 cups water (distilled). Cover skillet and simmer over low heat for 1 hour or until wild rice is light and fluffy. When done, let it remain covered for about 15 minutes, then fold pimento and parsley in wild rice mixture. Serve hot. Serves 8 to 10.

● ● ●

WILD RICE BROTH BAKE

1 Cup wild rice, raw
1/2 Lb. mushrooms
1/2 Cup celery, chopped
1 1/4 cups broth
1 Tablespoon butter
1/2 Cup onion, chopped

Wash wild rice; place in six-cup casserole. Cover with broth. Add onions and celery. Soak 3 hours. Saute mushrooms in butter. Add to wild rice and bake at least one hour, adding liquid if too dry. Serves 6 to 8.

BAKED STEAK STUFFED WITH WILD RICE

2 1/2 Cups wild rice, precooked
3 Tablespoons unbleached flour
1 1/2 Teaspoon sea salt
1/8 Teaspoon cayenne
1 1/2 Lbs. round steak, cut 1 inch thick
3 Tablespoons raw butter
1/2 Cup tomato juice
3/4 Cup water (distilled)
2 Tablespoons cold pressed oil
1/4 Cup onions, finely chopped

Combine 2 tablespoons flour, 1 teaspoon salt, and cayenne. Pound into meat on both sides. Saute chopped onions in butter until soft. Stir in remaining 1 tablespoon flour and 1/2 teaspoon salt. Add tomato juice and 1/4 cup water. Cook over low heat, stirring constantly until thickened. Add wild rice and blend. Spread mixture on steak. Roll and fasten with skewers. Brown meat well in oil. Add rest of water. Bake covered in 350 degree oven for 2 hours or until meat is tender. If desired, garnish with sauteed mushrooms. Serves 4 to 6.

SAFFRON WILD RICE

1/2 Cup wild rice, raw
2 Tablespoons raw butter
2 Tablespoons onion, chopped
1/16 Teaspoon ground saffron

Precook wild rice. Melt butter and saffron in skillet, add onion and cook until transparent. Blend precooked wild rice with onion mixture. Serves 4.

WILD RICE WITH NUTS AND HERBS

1/4 Cup wild rice, raw
1/2 Teaspoon sea salt
3 Cups cold water (distilled) or chicken (without skin) broth
1 Medium onion, chopped fine
1/4 Cup celery, minced
1/2 Cup broken walnuts, pine nuts or slivered almonds
1 Tablespoon parsley, chopped
1/2 Teaspoon dried rosemary
1/4 Teaspoon marjoram
1 1/2 Tablespoon raw butter

Wash wild rice in several waters and let soak in water an hour or so. Drain. Place in saucepan with salt and water or chicken broth. Bring to a boil and simmer, covered, until tender but not mushy. Drain and place in buttered casserole. Saute onions and celery in hot butter until tender. Add nuts and herbs and stir lightly into rice. Check seasoning and add salt if necessary. Cover and bake 15 minutes in 325 degree oven. Stir with fork to release steam. Rice should be fluffy and somewhat moist. If you need more seasoning, sprinkle with Vegit before serving. Serves 6 to 7.

7 LAYER DINNER

1 Layer potatoes, uncooked and sliced
1 Layer chopped onions
1 Layer wild rice, precooked 15 minutes
1 Layer carrots, sliced
1/2 Green pepper, chopped
1 Lb. very lean ground beef (optional)
2 Cups tomato sauce

Layer in deep casserole in order above. Season each layer.
Bake at 350 degrees for 1 1/2 to 2 hours or until potatoes
are done. Water may be needed to keep moist while
cooking. Serves 8.

WILD RICE MEAT BALLS

1/4 Cup wild rice, precooked or pureed
1 Lb. very lean ground beef
1 1/2 Cups pureed tomatoes
1 Egg, slightly beaten
2 Tablespoons parsley
1 Teaspoon sea salt
1/4 Teaspoon garlic powder
2 Tablespoons cold pressed oil
1 Cup water (distilled)
1/2 Cup onion, minced

Mix ground beef, one-fourth tomatoes, wild rice, egg,
parsley, onion and salt together. Shape into balls and
brown in skillet with garlic powder and oil. Mix together
remaining tomatoes and water. Add sauce and meatballs in
skillet and simmer covered 1 hour. Stir gently several times
and add more water if needed. Serves 4 to 6.

HIS FAVORITE CASSEROLE

1/2 Cup wild rice, raw
1/2 Cup brown rice, raw
1 1/3 Cups chicken (without skin) broth, thickened with
   2 tablespoons unbleached flour
1 Cup celery, chopped
1 Large onion, diced
3 Tablespoons soy sauce
1 Lb. very lean ground beef

Precook wild rice and brown rice. Brown ground beef and add onion, celery, soy sauce, broth and water (distilled). Mix thoroughly. Stir in drained rice. Bake in shallow pan 35 to 40 minutes at 375 degrees. Serves 6 to 8.

● ● ●

QUICK CASSEROLE

2 Cups chicken (without skin), cooked and diced
   (skin removed before cooking)
2 Tablespoons onion, diced
2 Cups wild rice, precooked
1 1/3 Cup homemade cream of celery soup

Mix all ingredients and place in shallow baking pan. Bake about 30 minutes in a 350 degree oven. Serves 4 to 6.

EASY HOT POT DINNER DISH

1/2 Cup wild rice, raw
1 Cup brown rice, raw
1 1/2 Lbs. very lean ground beef
1 Small onion, chopped
1 1/2 Cups tomato sauce
1 Teaspoon sea salt
1 Cup tomatoes pureed
1 1/2 Cup celery, chopped
Optional:
1 Tablespoon green pepper
1 Cup carrots, chopped
1 Cup peas (add last 15 minutes)

Preheat 3-quart Hot Pot to 300 degrees. Brown ground beef with onion, celery, and green pepper. Add remaining ingredients, except peas, and 3 cups hot water (distilled). Season with cayenne and more salt if needed. Simmer 1 1/2 to 2 hours. Serves 6 to 8.

WHOLE WILD RICE MUFFINS

1 Cup wild rice, precooked
1 1/2 Cups flour, unbleached
3 Tablespoons cold pressed oil
1/2 Teaspoon sea salt
1 1/2 Tablespoons honey
1 Teaspoon baking powder
1 Egg, beaten
1 Cup non-fat milk

Sift dry ingredients. Cut in oil. Add wild rice, egg, honey, and milk. Mix and divide mixture into 12 muffin pans. Bake at 425 degrees for 20 minutes. Makes 12 muffins.

WILD RICE MUFFINS

1/4 Cup wild rice flour
1 1/4 cups sifted unbleached flour
3 Teaspoons baking powder
1 Teaspoon sea salt
1/4 Cup honey
1 Egg
1 Large tablespoon honey
1 Cup non-fat milk
1/4 cup cold pressed oil

Sift together flour, baking powder, salt, and wild rice flour. Add to well-beaten mixture of eggs, milk, honey, and oil. Do not over mix. Pour into well-greased muffin pans. Bake in 400 degree oven about 15 minutes or until muffins are golden brown. Makes 10 to 12 muffins.

Breads

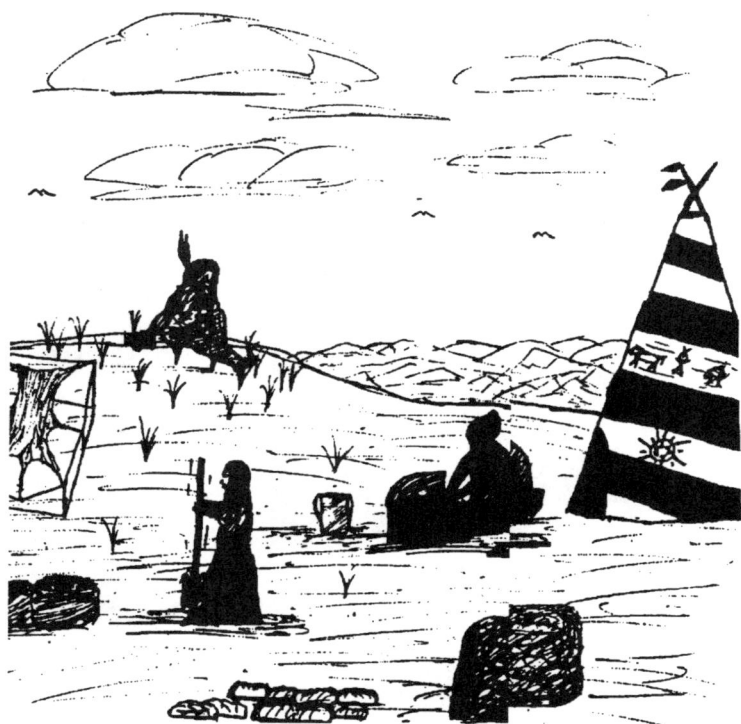

BREADS

Everyone has always loved homemade bread. Now we have an excuse to have it every day. But what about those days when there's no bread made and no time to make it? All health food stores have whole grain breads without additives or preservatives. There are also several brands in the supermarkets that adhere to our diet. Orowheat Wheat Berry bread is very delicious; also Granola and Branola. Pita or Bible bread is also available in health food stores.

A helpful hint when cooking breads with whole grain flour is to add either 1/2 teaspoon granulated or 1 crushed 500 ml. Vitamin C tablet to the dry ingredients. For some unknown reason it causes it to rise and be lighter and fluffier.

There are also several brands of automatic bread makers on the market. They come with recipe books that are very easily modified to our diet. I love mine because I can just throw all the ingredients in the night before (takes about 5 minutes), set the automatic timer and then I wake up the next morning to the smell of freshly baked bread.

POCKET BREAD

Pocket Bread, Pita Bread, or Bible Bread are three names given to a most unique food that is becoming more and more popular in the United States. It is a round flat bread that parts in the middle and makes a 'pocket' that you can fill with all sorts of goodies. Pocket Bread is the bread mentioned in the Bible and is the native bread of the Middle East.

It can be bought frozen in most health food stores or you can easily make it yourself. There is no end to the variations of the uses of pocket bread. Just as you can let your imagination run wild with juices, drinks, herbs, and sprouts, you can do unlimited things with pocket bread. After two years I am still finding new ways to stuff it.

I am including both the recipe for making the bread along with a few suggestions on serving. Try these and then experiment on your own.

1 Tablespoon yeast
1 1/2 Cups lukewarm water
3 to 4 Cups whole wheat flour

Have the water warm but not hot. Dissolve yeast in water. Stir in 2 cups flour. Beat vigorously at least 2 minutes to add air and develop the gluten. Add the rest of the flour 1/2 cup at a time until the dough forms a ball firm enough to knead.

Knead the dough on a lightly floured board until smooth and elastic and no longer sticks to your fingers. Separate the dough into two inch balls. Roll out on lightly floured board to one-fourth inch. Being perfectly round is not as important as having the dough a uniform thickness.

Let rise for 45 minutes. Preheat oven to 500 degrees. I know that sounds too hot, but it is the right temperature. Place circles on ungreased cookie sheet and bake 5 minutes, turn circles over and bake for five more minutes.

Use amounts of ingredients according to the number of sandwiches you plan to serve - one or twenty.

AVOCADO PITA

Mash avocado and add homemade mayonnaise and a few drops of lemon juice. Stuff in bottom of pockets. Add some shredded lettuce, chopped tomato, and chopped onion and top with a little cottage cheese. Add some salsa in the lettuce for seasoning. You may use any kind of sprouts in place of the lettuce.

SPROUT AND BEAN PITA

Stuff mashed pinto beans in pocket first. Then add alfalfa sprouts, salsa, or Spike (or both).

EGG PITA

Dry fry an egg. Tilt the skillet around on all sides to spread the egg out. Break the middle so it mixes with the white. Gently slide the egg into the pocket. Stuff sprouts, cottage cheese seasoned with Vegit, Spike, garlic salt, kelp, or anything you can think of that tastes good to you.

HINTS FOR PITA VARIATIONS

Stuff the pocket first with mashed pinto beans then add mashed avocado seasoned with your favorite herb, a few drops of lemon juice. Add a little shredded lettuce or sprouts.

Mix mashed pinto beans and cottage cheese together and stuff in pocket. Add some salsa and sprouts or lettuce.

Mix cooked lentils with mashed banana and stuff in pocket. Add chopped lettuce and tomatoes. I know a mixture of lentils and bananas may sound strange to you, but they are delicious.

● ● ●

WHOLE WHEAT BISCUITS

1 3/4 Cups whole wheat flour
3/4 Teaspoon sea salt
2 1/2 Teaspoons baking powder
3 Tablespoons cold pressed oil
1 Cup milk (non-fat)
1/2 Teaspoon granulated Vitamin C

Mix dry ingredients. Pour oil in milk and add to dry ingredients. Stir well and place on floured board. Sprinkle with flour and pat out to one-half inch thick. Cut with biscuit cutter. Place in greased pan and bake at 450 degrees until brown on top.

HINT: Add 1/2 teaspoon granulated Vitamin C or one 500 milligram Vitamin C tablet, crushed, to whole wheat bread recipes and they will be much fluffier. Don't ask why. Someone told me to try it, I did, and it worked!!

SOURDOUGH STARTER

For best results use glass or pottery containers. Never use a metal container or leave a metal spoon in the starter. A good starter contains only flour, water, and yeast. It has a clean sour milk odor. The liquid will separate from the batter when it stands several days, but this does not matter. If replenished every few days with flour and more water, the starter keeps fresh. If starter is not to be used for several weeks, freeze or dry it to keep from spoiling. To carry it to camp, add enough flour to shape it into a ball and place it in a sack of flour. In the dried form the yeast goes into a spore state which will keep inert for a long time like old-fashioned yeast foam. Water and warmth bring the yeast back to the active stage.

2 Cups unbleached flour
2 Cups warm water
1 Package dry yeast

Place ingredients in a warm place or closed cupboard overnight. In the morning put cup of the starter in a scalded pint jar with a tight cover and store in the refrigerator or cool place for future use. This is sourdough starter. The remaining batter can be used for pancakes, waffles, muffins, bread, or cake immediately.

HONEY BRAN MUFFINS

2 Cups sifted unbleached flour
4 Teaspoons baking powder
3/4 Teaspoon sea salt
2 Cups bran
1 Tablespoon raw butter
3/4 Cup mixed, chopped almonds and sunflower seeds
1 Well beaten egg
1/2 Cup raw honey
1 1/4 Cups non-fat milk
1/2 Teaspoon Vitamin C

Sift flour, baking powder and salt. Stir in the bran and nut with seeds. Add rest of ingredients stirring only until mixed. Fill oiled muffin pans 2/3 full and bake at 425 degrees for 25 to 35 minutes. About 16 large muffins.

● ● ●

RYE MUFFINS

Combine and mix well:
1 Cup whole rye flour
2 Teaspoons honey

1/2 Teaspoon sea salt
1 Teaspoon baking
powder

Blend and mix well:
1/4 Cup non-fat milk
1 Teaspoon cold pressed oil

1 Well beaten egg

Fold into dry ingredients. Bake at 350 degrees in well oiled muffin tins for 25 minutes. Makes 6 large muffins.

BASIC COARSE TEXTURED FRENCH BREAD

2 1/2 Cups very warm water (distilled)
2 Packages dry yeast
6 Cups unsifted unbleached flour
2 Teaspoons sea salt
2 Teaspoons water (distilled)

Sprinkle yeast over water in large bowl; stir to dissolve. Let stand about 5 minutes.

Add 3 1/2 to 4 cups of flour, 1/2 cup at a time, beating with electric mixer, until a smooth batter forms. (If beaters become strained, stir in remaining flour.) Beat batter at least 10 minutes to develop gluten. Dissolve salt in 2 teaspoons water; add to batter. Blend in. Stir enough of the remaining in to form a soft dough. Knead on floured board 7 or 8 minutes, using only enough flour to keep dough from sticking.

Place dough in greased bowl, cover with plastic wrap and let rise 2 hours. Punch down, knead briefly in bowl. Re-cover and let rise 1 1/2 hours.

Place dough on lightly floured surface and divide into 4 pieces. Shape each piece to a 16 to 18 inch length, tapered at ends. Transfer to two large cookie sheets. Let rise till more than double. Make diagonal cuts on top with razor blade or very sharp knife.

Preheat oven to 450 degrees. Place a shallow pan on bottom shelf. Five minutes before baking, carefully pour 1 cup water into hot pan to create steam for baking. Bake loaves on middle shelf about 25 minutes, or until brown and loaves sound hollow when tapped. Cool on wire rack. Does this sound like too much trouble? If so buy a bread maker and follow the recipe.

REFRIGERATOR PAN ROLLS

Combine:
3/4 Cup hot water (distilled)
1/3 Cup raw honey
1 Tablespoon sea salt
3 Tablespoons unsalted raw butter

Dissolve 2 packages dry yeast in one cup water. Add to water mixture.

Add:
1 Beaten egg
2 1/2 Cups unbleached flour

Beat until smooth.

Add enough unbleached flour (about 2 3/4 cups) to make a soft dough.

Turn out on lightly floured board; knead until smooth and elastic. Place in greased bowl, turning to grease top. Cover tightly. Store in refrigerator at least 2 hours or overnight. Turn out on floured board, punch down. Make into rolls. Let rise one hour. Bake at 375 degrees for 20 minutes or until brown on top.

SOUTHERN CORN BREAD

1 1/4 cups stone ground corn meal
3/4 cup whole wheat flour
2 1/2 Teaspoons baking powder
1 Teaspoon sea salt
1 Egg
1 1/4 Cups non-fat milk
1/4 Cup cold pressed oil

Mix all ingredients except oil. Heat oil in skillet and pour into batter. Mix well and pour into hot skillet. Bake at 450 degrees till brown on top.

If you like crispy bread, sprinkle cornmeal in the bottom of an iron skillet and pour mixture on top. Of course you realize I'm talking about an old iron skillet like grandmother used. If you don't have one, buy one at the Goodwill store and enjoy old-fashioned cornbread.

● ● ●

QUICK ROLLS

1 Cup non-fat milk
1 Package dry yeast
2 Tablespoons cold pressed oil
1 Tablespoon raw honey
1 1/2 Cups whole wheat flour
1 1/2 Cups unbleached flour
1/2 Teaspoon granulated Vitamin C

Mix ingredients well. If dough seems too stiff add a little more milk. Set in warm place for about 30 minutes or until dough rises. Work down, pat dough out thin, cut with biscuit cutter, dip in melted butter, place in pan in warm place until rolls rise double. Bake at 450 degrees until done.

CRANBERRY NUT BREAD

2 Cups unbleached flour
2/3 Cup raw honey
1 1/2 Teaspoons baking powder
1/2 Teaspoon sea salt
1/2 Teaspoon soda
1/4 Cup cold pressed oil
1 Teaspoon grated orange peel
3/4 Cup orange juice
1 Well beaten egg
1 Cup coarsely chopped cranberries
1/2 Cup chopped nuts

Sift dry ingredients. Add oil. Combine peel, juice, and egg. Add to mixture, just to moisten. Fold in berries and nuts. Cook in greased 9x5x3 inch pan. Bake at 350 degrees for 1 hour. Cool - wrap - store overnight.

You can use whole wheat flour and 1/2 teaspoon granulated Vitamin C to make this bread.

MILLET BY TRISH COTTER

Cook millet only until chewy*
    (do not overcook)
Add 1 tablespoon olive oil
    Raw scallions (green onions)
    Raw garlic
    Kelp (to taste)

Combine 1 glass raw goat's milk and you have a biologically superior protein, compared to animal protein, which will help the body rather than harm, as does animal protein. Serves 1.
*Such as you do with brown rice.

184

GRANOLA CRACKERS

2 Cups rolled oats
3/4 Cup whole wheat flour
1/2 Cup slivered almonds
1/4 Cup wheat germ
1/4 Cup sesame seeds
3/4 Teaspoon sea salt
1 Tablespoon honey
1/2 Teaspoon leaf oregano, crumbled
1 Teaspoon leaf thyme, crumbled
1/2 Teaspoon onion powder
3 Eggs
3/4 Cup vegetable oil

Combine oats, flour, almonds, wheat germ, sesame seeds, honey, salt, oregano, thyme and onion powder in large bowl. In small bowl beat: eggs and oil until well mixed. Stir into oat mixture till well blended. Spread mixture into well greased 15x10x1 inch jelly roll pan. Level top with spatula. Bake in pre-heated oven 400 degrees for 20 minutes. (Air bubbles will subside on top when removed from oven.) Remove pan to wire rack. Cut squares of 1 1/2 inches, then cut in 1/2 to make triangles. When cool, store in tightly covered container. Cracker will keep for several weeks in the refrigerator. Makes 1 1/2 pounds.

SOFT BREAD STICKS

1/2 Cup very warm water (distilled)
1 Envelope active dry yeast
2 Tablespoons honey
1/2 Cup (1 stick) unsalted raw butter (melted)
1 Teaspoon sea salt
1/2 Cup boiling water (distilled)
1 Egg
2 to 2 1/2 Cups whole wheat flour
1/2 Teaspoon water (distilled)
Caraway or sesame seeds

Sprinkle yeast over very warm water in a 1 cup measure.
(water should feel comfortably warm when dropped on
wrist.) Stir in 1 teaspoon of honey. Let stand until bubbly,
about 10 minutes. Mix salt, butter, boiling water and
remaining honey in a large bowl; cool till lukewarm. Beat
egg in a small cup, reserve 1 tablespoon for brushing sticks.
Stir remaining egg into butter mixture. Stir in yeast until
blended. Add 2 cups of flour; gradually stir in enough extra
flour to make a soft dough. Do not knead. Divide dough
into 12 parts. Roll each on floured surface to make an even
stick 12 inches long. On greased cookie sheet place about
2 inches apart. Mix reserved egg with the 1/2 teaspoon of
water. Brush over bread sticks and sprinkle with seeds. Let
stand, uncovered for 30 minutes.

Bake in a hot oven 425 degrees for 15 minutes. Remove to
wire rack and serve warm. For shorter sticks divide dough
into 24 parts.

HONEY WHOLE WHEAT BREAD

5 Cups warm water (110° F) distilled
2 Packages active dry yeast
6 Tablespoons cold pressed oil
1/4 Cup honey
4 Cups whole wheat flour
1/2 Cup instant potatoes*
1/2 Cup instant dry milk
2 Teaspoons sea salt
6 1/2 to 8 Cups unbleached flour

Combine 1/2 cup water and yeast in a small bowl, stir to dissolve yeast. In a large container, mix oil, honey, and remaining water. Mix whole wheat flour, instant potatoes, dry milk and salt. Add to water mixture and beat until smooth. Add yeast mixture and beat until smooth. Then with a wooden spoon mix in enough unbleached flour to make a dough that cleans the pan. Knead on lightly floured board until smooth and elastic, about 8 to 10 minutes. Place in greased bowl; turn dough so top is greased. Cover; let rise in warm place until doubled, 1 to 1 1/2 hours. Punch down dough; divide in thirds; cover and let rest 5 minutes. Shape into 3 loaves. Place in greased pans (9x5x3); brush tops with cold pressed oil. Cover; let rise until doubled, about 1 hour. Bake in 400 degree oven about 50 minutes. Remove from pans; cool on rack. May be packaged and frozen when cool.

*NOTE: May use 1 cup mashed potatoes in place of instant mashed. Combine with the honey-water mixture.

WHEAT GERM PANCAKES

1/2 Cup warm water (distilled)
2 Tablespoons dry yeast
2 Tablespoons honey
1 Cup whole wheat flour
1 Cup wheat germ
1 Cup non-fat milk
2 Tablespoons cold pressed oil

Combine yeast, honey and water in bowl and let rise for 30 minutes. Add remaining ingredients and mix well. Cook on moderately hot griddle.

● ● ●

QUICK LOAF OF BREAD

2 1/2 Cups whole wheat flour
1 Teaspoon baking soda
1 Teaspoon sea salt
1 Teaspoon baking powder
Pinch of cinnamon

Sift together and add:
1/2 Cup raw honey
1/4 Cup cold pressed oil
1 1/2 Cups buttermilk
1/2 Cup chopped raw walnuts
1 Tablespoon grated orange rind

Stir together and pour into loaf pan. Let stand 20 minutes, then bake at 375 degrees for 45 to 60 minutes, until brown on top and toothpick comes out clean.

GRAIN, NUT, FRUIT CEREAL

3 Cups raw, rolled oats
1/2 Cup wheat germ
1 1/2 Cups unsweetened shredded coconut
1/4 Cup sesame seeds
1/2 Cup wheat germ
1/2 Cup raw honey
1/4 Cup cold pressed oil
1/2 Cup cold distilled water
1 Cup slivered almonds
1/2 Cup sun dried raisins

Preheat oven to 250 degrees.

Combine first five ingredients in large bowl. Combine honey and oil. Mix together and stir until well blended. Add water a little at a time and stir till crumbly.

Place mixture into large, shallow baking pan that is lightly oiled. Bake for two hours, stirring every 15 minutes. Add the almonds and bake one half hour longer. Cool in oven. Add raisins. Store tightly covered in a cool, dry place. Serve covered with apple juice.

Sweets

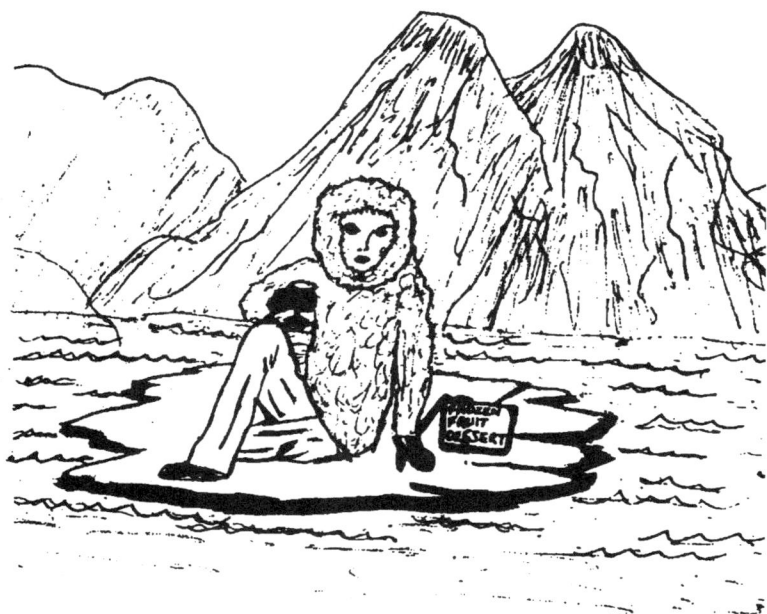

SWEETS

Even though we have included this chapter on sweets, they should be eaten sparingly. A good diet of fresh fruits, fresh vegetables, and whole grains is still the best insurance for good nutrition.

If you feel you must have something sweet occasionally, these recipes have been designed to fall within the limits of our diet.

PLAIN 2 EGG CAKE

2 Cups whole wheat pastry flour
2 1/2 Teaspoon baking powder
1 Teaspoon sea salt
1/2 Cup cold pressed oil
1/2 Cup raw honey
1 Cup non-fat milk
2 Eggs
2 Teaspoons pure vanilla
1/2 Teaspoon granulated Vitamin C

Mix dry ingredients. Beat in oil, honey, and half the milk for 2 minutes at medium speed of mixer. Add rest of ingredients and beat again. Bake in ungreased 9 x 13 inch pan for 35 minutes at 350 degrees. Serve with apple syrup, yogurt icing or walnut icing.

● ● ●

WALNUT ICING

2/3 Cup non-fat milk
1/4 Cup raw honey
2 Teaspoons whole wheat flour
1 Cup finely chopped walnuts

Mix milk, honey, and flour in small pan and cook over low heat till thick, stirring constantly. Stir in nuts. Pour over Plain Cake.

MUSHROOM SAUCE

1/2 Cup sliced mushrooms
2 Tablespoons unsalted raw butter
2 Tablespoons unbleached flour
3/4 Cup chicken (without skin) broth
1/2 Cup non-fat milk

Saute mushrooms in oil. Mix flour and chicken broth and add to mushrooms. Slowly add milk. Serve over vegetables.

CAROB BROWNIES

1 Cup sifted whole wheat flour
1 Teaspoon baking powder
1/4 Teaspoon sea salt
1/2 Cup raw butter
1/2 cup carob powder
1 Cup honey
2 Eggs, well beaten
1/2 Cup chopped walnuts
1 Teaspoon pure vanilla

Sift first 3 ingredients and set aside. Melt butter in small saucepan over low heat. Add carob powder and honey and blend. Remove from heat. Beat eggs well and add carob mixture. Add dry ingredients and mix well. Stir in vanilla and nuts. Spread into oiled 8 inch square pan. Bake at 350 degrees for 40 minutes or until toothpick comes out clean when inserted in center. Cool before cutting into squares.

BAKED BANANAS

4 Medium bananas
1 Tablespoon unsalted raw butter
1 Tablespoon raw honey
1 Teaspoon lemon juice
1/2 Teaspoon grated lemon peel

Arrange halved, peeled bananas in oiled baking dish. Sprinkle with mixture of butter, honey, lemon juice and peel. Bake at 350 degrees for 15 to 20 minutes. Serve as a dessert or side dish with chicken.

CHRISTMAS FRUIT CAKE

1/2 Cup sunflower, sesame, or cold pressed oil
2/3 Cup raw honey
3 Well beaten eggs
1 Tablespoon each lemon and orange rind
2 1/2 Cups whole wheat flour
1/4 Teaspoon kelp powder
1/4 Teaspoon allspice
1 Cup each of raisins and walnuts
1 Teaspoon baking powder
1/4 Cup fresh orange juice
1/2 Cup each of 3 dried unsulphured fruits
    (i.e., apricot, apple, peach)

Sift dry ingredients and slowly mix in other ingredients. Mix well. Pour into oiled and floured 9x5x3 inch loaf pan and bake at 325 degrees for 1 1/2 hours.

FRUIT SHERBET

1 1/2 Cups fresh orange juice
3/4 Cup lemon juice
3 Medium bananas
3 Cups cold water (distilled)
2 Cups non-fat milk
1 Tablespoon honey

Blend for 2 minutes on high speed. Pour in mold and freeze.

FROZEN FRUIT DESSERT

3/4 Cup fresh lemon, lime, or orange juice
Grated lemon, lime, or orange peel
4 Cups water
2 Teaspoons honey

Mix well and put in freezer tray. Freeze until barely firm. Break into chunks. Repeat several times. Heap into small bowls. Frozen raspberries or blueberries pureed in blender makes a beautiful sauce. Just pour over each serving.

● ● ●

YOGURT ICE CREAM

2 Cups plain natural unsweetened yogurt
2 Cups finely chopped fresh fruit
Raw honey to taste

Mix all ingredients and spread in ice tray and freeze.

● ● ●

PIE DOUGH

2 1/2 Cups whole wheat flour
1/2 Teaspoon sea salt
1/3 Cup cold pressed oil
1/3 Cup water (distilled)

Mix lightly with fork. Roll out 1/2 of dough between waxed paper. Bake at 375 degrees till done - about 15 minutes.

HONEY COOKIES

1/2 Cup cold pressed oil
1/2 Cup raw honey
1 Well beaten egg
2 Teaspoons pure vanilla
1 Cup whole wheat flour

Mix all liquids. Stir in flour. You should have a stiff dough. If not add a little more flour. Drop by teaspoonfuls on oiled cookie sheet. Bake 12 -15 minutes at 375 degrees or till edges are brown.

● ● ●

BROILED GRAPEFRUIT

2 Large grapefruit - halves
2 Tablespoons raw butter
2 Teaspoons honey
1/2 Cup cinnamon - honey mixture
    (1 part cinnamon to 4 parts honey)

Make sure grapefruit halves are room temperature. Cut around each section of each half. Sections should be completely loosened from shell. Cut hole in center of each half, fill with butter. Spread with honey and then honey mixture.

QUICK PRUNE DESSERT

4 Egg whites
3/4 Cup pureed prunes
2 1/2 Teaspoons lemon juice

Beat egg whites till stiff. Fold in prunes and lemon juice. Chill.

SWEET CRUMB CRUST

1 Cup crushed honey cookies
1/2 Cup wheat germ
1/3 Cup cold pressed oil

Mix all ingredients. Press in pie plate. Chill.

Fill with carob tapioca or rice pudding or custard. This is very good for the family. Laetrile users, only a small portion! Once.

CHUNKY APPLESAUCE

Pare, core, and slice 4 medium applies. Combine 1 cup water, 1/4 cup honey and a dash of mace and bring to a boil. Add apples, cover and simmer till tender for 8 minutes.

● ● ●

BAKED APPLES

4 Cups sliced pared tart apples
1/4 Cup fresh orange juice
1 Cup honey
3/4 Cup sifted whole wheat flour
1/2 Teaspoon ground cinnamon
1/4 Teaspoon ground nutmeg
1/2 Cup raw butter

Place apples in greased (with butter) 9-inch pie plate. Combine honey, flour, spices; cut in butter till mixed. Spread over apples. Bake at 375 degrees for 45 minutes or till apples are tender. Serve warm. 6 servings. Broil 4 inches from heat 8 to 10 minutes or till tops are brown. Serves 4.

MERINGUE

Beat 2 egg whites till frothy. Add 1/2 cup water (distilled) very slowly and beat till stiff. Gradually beat in 2 teaspoon honey. Spread on custard and bake at 325 degrees for 15 minutes or till brown on top.

● ● ●

CUSTARD VARIATIONS

Chocolate - add 2 teaspoons carob powder

Fruit Cream Pies - add 2 cups fresh fruit of any kind to custard and top with meringue.

APRICOT BROWNIES

1 1/2 Cup dried apricots
2 Cups distilled water
4 Tablespoons raw honey
1 1/2 Cups rolled oats
1 1/2 Cups whole wheat flour
1/2 Cup chopped pecans
1/2 Cup cold pressed oil
1/2 Cup raw honey

Mix apricots, water, and honey in pan. Simmer over low heat for 10 minutes. Mix oats, flour, nuts, oil, and honey. Press half of mixture in bottom of 8x8-inch pan. Spread fruit mixture on top. Sprinkle remaining oat mixture over top. Bake at 350 degrees for 20 to 30 minutes or till lightly browned. Cool before cutting.

OATMEAL COOKIES

1 Tablespoon cold pressed oil
1/2 Cup raw honey
2 Beaten eggs
1/2 Teaspoon sea salt
2 Cups rolled oats
1/2 Cup whole wheat flour
1 Tablespoon grated lemon rind

Mix all ingredients to make a stiff dough. If it seems too thick, add a little non-fat milk. Drop by teaspoonsful on oiled cookie sheet. Bake at 400 degrees for 8 to 10 minutes.

CUSTARD

1 3/4 Cups non-fat milk
2 Egg yolks
1/4 Cup unbleached flour
2/3 Cup honey

Mix 1/2 cup milk with flour. Stir in egg yolks and honey. Gradually add rest of milk. Cook over low flame stirring constantly till thick. Pour into prepared shell.

YOGURT DIP

1/2 Cup plain natural yogurt
4 Tablespoons raw honey
1/3 Cup non-fat milk powder
1 Tablespoon vanilla
Juice of 1/2 lime

Blend all ingredients. Chill. Add a little unsweetened apple juice before serving if it gets too thick. Prepare a platter of chunks of fresh fruit. Use toothpicks to spear fruit and dip. When using banana or apple chunks, remember to coat with lemon or lime juice to prevent darkening.

● ● ●

YOGURT ICING

Prepare yogurt dip and add 1 tablespoon raw butter and more milk powder to make it thick and creamy.

For fruit filling, add any crushed fresh fruit.

FRUIT COBBLER

6 Tablespoons unsalted raw butter
1 1/2 Cups whole wheat flour
1/4 Teaspoon sea salt
1 Teaspoon baking powder
1/2 Cup raw honey
1 Beaten egg
1 Cup non-fat milk
2 Cups any fresh fruit

(For extra tart fruit, add 1/4 cup more honey.) Preheat oven to 400 degrees. Melt butter in 1 1/2 quart flat stainless steel pan or glass baking dish. Mix flour, salt, baking powder, honey, egg, and milk. Pour over butter. Do not stir. Pour fruit on top. Do not stir. Bake 30 to 35 minutes. Dough will come to the top and brown.

TAPIOCA WITH CAROB

2 Eggs
6 Tablespoons tapioca
1/4 Cup honey
3 Cups non-fat milk
1/4 Cup sifted carob powder
1/4 Cup boiling water (distilled)
1 Teaspoon pure vanilla

Break eggs in saucepan and beat lightly with a fork. Add tapioca and honey. Add milk. Mix carob with boiling water until dissolved. Add to mixture and cook over moderate heat, stirring constantly, until pudding boils. Let stand 15 minutes before stirring in vanilla. Pour into dessert dishes and chill.

FRESH APPLE CAKE

1 1/4 Cups cold pressed oil
1 1/3 Cups raw honey
3 Cups unbleached flour
2 Eggs
1 Teaspoon soda
1 Teaspoon cinnamon
1/2 Teaspoon salt
3 Cups diced raw apples
1 Cup pecans

Dredge apples and pecans in one cup of the flour and set aside to add last. Mix oil and sugar together, add eggs and mix. Mix in the two remaining cups of flour along with soda, salt, and cinnamon, then stir in the apple, nut, and flour mixture. (Dough will be very stiff.) Bake in lightly oiled 9x13 inch pan at 350 degrees for 40 to 50 minutes or until done.

● ● ●

RICE PUDDING

1 1/2 Cups cooked brown rice
1 1/2 Cups non-fat milk
1 Egg, beaten
2 Tablespoons raw honey
1/2 Cup raisins
2 Teaspoon lemon rind
Dash of sea salt
Dash of ground cinnamon
1/2 Cup chopped pecans (optional)

Mix all ingredients except nuts and cook over low heat for 20 minutes. Add a little more honey to taste. Stir in pecans. Serve hot or cold.

DATE COOKIES

1 Cup whole wheat flour
1/2 Teaspoon granulated Vitamin C
3 Cups rolled oats
1 Cup chopped pecans
1 Cup chopped dates
1/4 Teaspoon sea salt
1/4 Cup cold pressed oil
1 Cup apple juice

Brown flour lightly in pan over low flame, stirring constant-ly. When cool, mix in all the dry ingredients. Add dates and nuts. Stir in oil and apple juice. Roll dough into small balls. (If dough is too sticky to roll, add more flour. If it is too dry, add more liquid.) Place on oiled cookie sheet. Flatten each cookie with a fork. Bake at 350 degrees for 20 to 30 minutes.

I hope that you have found this book to be helpful in helping you to live a more healthful lifestyle. I have tried to include recipes for anyone who wants to learn better ways to prepare foods and also to know the best foods to eat whether or not you are a vegetarian.

I will be happy to hear from you as to your feelings about this book and any suggestions you may have for future printings. So much new information becomes available every day, we are already working on the update for this book to have it ready for the next printing. For that reason, I will be anxious to hear from you.

For updates on this book, other new recipes we have discovered, new appliances on the market, regular copies of our FREE NEWSLETTER, or any questions or suggestions you may have please write to me at the following address:

PATRICIA PRINCE
RT.3, BOX 297
MEXIA, TEXAS 76667

ORDER FORM

NAME . . . .

ADDRESS . . . .

CITY . . . . ZIP . . . . . .

COMMENTS: . . . .

. . . .

. . . .

. . . .

. . . .

. . . .

TO ORDER PLEASE PRINT NAME AND ADDRESS. YOUR COMMENTS ARE GREATLY APPRECIATED.

INDEX

INDEX

INDEX

INDEX

INDEX

INDEX

INDEX

INDEX

INDEX

INDEX

Notes:

Notes: